# DO I CALL THE VET ?

## and what to do in the meantime

**Dr. Richard Chapman BVSc**

DISCLAIMER

This book is based on my experience, but is only intended for general information, and does not replace consultation with, or advice from, the veterinary practitioner or other health care professional involved with animals.

COPYRIGHT

Copyright © 2015 Dr. R.H.Chapman BVSc

The right of R.H.Chapman to be identified as the author of this work has been asserted by him in accordance with the Copyright, Designs and Patents Act 1988.

Published by Touchworks Ltd. a company registered in England, United Kingdom No. 03668464.
Registered Office: 67 London Road, St Leonards-on-Sea, East Sussex TN37 6AR

Available in print and as an e-book from Amazon and www.lulu.com

A catalogue record for this title is available from the British Library.

# ABOUT THE AUTHOR

Dr. Richard Chapman is a very experienced veterinarian. Over the years, he has worked both in mixed practice, as the equine expert, and in sole practice. In addition to conventional veterinary science, he has studied holistic and alternative medicine, natural medicine and folk or 'bush' remedies.

Dr. Chapman has enjoyed participating in many equine modalities including pleasure, sporting and stud work. In particular, he worked very closely with endurance riding from its commencement in Australia, helping to establish the sport from 1975 onwards, and holding the post of its ACT senior equine veterinary surgeon from 1975 to 1998.

He has held the following posts:

- *Official Veterinarian of ACT Racing Club 1975 — 2007*
- *Official Veterinarian of Canberra Harness Racing Club 1979 —2011*
- *Official Veterinarian of Queanbeyan Racing Club 1983 — 2000*
- *Member of the ACT Veterinary Surgeons Board 1993 —2004 of which he was chair for two years.*
- *Chief Veterinarian Royal National Capital Agricultural Society (Canberra Show) 1986 — 2006*
- *Chief Veterinarian Royal Agricultural Show (Sydney Royal Easter Show) 1987 —2004*
- *ACT District Endurance Riders Association Honorary Veterinarian 1982—2000*
- *Veterinary Team Member Quilty 160 Km Endurance Ride 1982—2000*

In 2007 he was awarded the Canberra Racing Club Trophy for Services to Horse Racing and the Australian Veterinary Association Meritorious Award.

Positions within the Australian Veterinary Association:

- *Committee Member and Past President of the ACT Division of the Australian Veterinary Association*
- *Deputy Convenor of the ACT Division of the Australian Veterinary Association Conference*
- *Council Member of the ACT Division of the Australian Veterinary Association*

Former memberships

- *Council Member of the Australian and New Zealand Veterinary Council*
- *The Australian Equine Veterinary Association*
- *The British Equine Veterinary Association*
- *The Australian Holistic Veterinary Association and*
- *The Australian Veterinary Acupuncturist Association.*

Currently Dr Chapman is a member of the *Australian Veterinary Association.*
Web: www.richardchapman.vet

# FOREWORD

I read Veterinary Science at Bristol University in England, completing my B.V.Sc. Degree, after five years hard slog, in 1958. Within three weeks of qualifying I started work as a Veterinary Surgeon in a very mixed practice in Kent, and I have practised as a veterinarian ever since. I calculate that now (2015) I have spent fifty-seven continuous years in practice.

I practised for nine of those years in various parts of England. The remaining years have been spent in Australia: the first eight in Orbost, Victoria, and the rest in Canberra. This means that I have been practising in Canberra for over forty years!

When I started work, veterinary practice was very different from the way it is today in 2015. We had none of today's diagnostic tools, such as ultrasound and X-rays, not to mention all the other lovely toys available now. Instead we had to hone our senses. We used our eyes; we had to develop brains in our fingertips so that we could 'feel' what was happening; we used our sense of smell; and we learned to listen to our intuition and experience. These arts are now almost dead.

Instead, veterinary hospitals abound and veterinarians can choose from a host of tests and a plethora of diagnostic tools. The unfortunate result, due to massive overheads, is that veterinary services are now very expensive — and unfortunately many people simply cannot afford them. The sad result is often that an ill animal either goes without treatment or is euthanised (put to sleep).

My philosophy is that there is both an art and a science to veterinary work. I believe that the animal's welfare comes first and attention to the owner's emotions comes a close second.

The purpose of this handbook is to pass on information that works. Much of the content is based on experience and the arts I have described. It is not a scientific manual, but a practical quick reference for home treatment. Of course, when thinking of and deciding upon treatment options, one must consider both art and science, together with the cost of treatment and the owners ability to provide veterinary nursing.

Lastly, this booklet contains my views only. If what I recommend is at odds with your own veterinarian's opinion, then you should take his or her advice, rather than rely upon this book.

*Richard H Chapman B.V.Sc*.
www.richardchapman.vet

# CONTENTS

# HORSES

# FEEDING and DIET

I will briefly touch on diet because I feel this has a basic effect on possible gut pathology. What I am about to say is very rudimentary and I do not intend to gainsay any dieticians' advice.

I tend to turn to nature for feeds. I have always thought the best veterinary advice is given by 'Dr. Green'. Horses in nature graze through the day, thus the stomach is seldom empty.

Horses kept stabled are usually fed twice a day, so at some stage the stomach is empty, allowing the digestive juices to act on the stomach lining and thus the animal is prone to get ulcers.

In Kentucky at one stage, all the paddocks were kept beautiful by being groomed so that they always looked lush. Believe it or not, a yearly figure of 2% of the horse population was afflicted with 'twist type' colic. An Irish veterinarian, managing one of the stables, spoilt the look of the scenery by putting in racks with hay. The rate of 'twist' became non-existent. The moral of this is that the horse requires *fibre* and of course in nature will pick whatever is available.

Performance horses, particularly those of the racing breeds, require more energy and hence are fed concentrates. Simply put, these are broken down in the higher gut to form propionic acid and *energy*. In cold weather most horses, and I'm now talking of pleasure horses in particular, will prefer hay or fibrous foods that are broken down in the large gut (colon) to acetic acid and *heat*.

## THE MOUTH

I intend to digress somewhat here, as the whole of an animal's welfare relates largely to this part of the body. A lot of nonsense is talked about keeping animals 'naturally' and nowhere is this truer than in the case of the horse. I am not going to consider other herbivores because they are usually left to their own devices.

However, the poor old horse is subjected to great abuse particularly from those who want things done 'naturally' with least apparent trauma to the horse. These people are, through what they think is kindness, being probably the most 'naturally' cruel of all.

In nature, a horse is a grazing animal. This means it has its head down eating 15 to 18 hours a day. Remember, head down — but an occasional forage higher. This represents 60,000 chews daily, not up and down but a rotational grind. They must do this to crush fibrous stalks, and whilst doing this the circular motion progressively rotates the food (stalks) to the more rear teeth which grind the material into smaller and smaller particles before being swallowed.

In our infinite kindness, we put these animals into a lush fenced area with too much food eaten too quickly. (This, of course, preconditions the horse to founder.) Then, bare paddocks and stalls, not much to eat for a lot of the day but, good hard feeds night and morning. This induces ulcers because feed is not in the stomach all the time, and thus acid works on the lining of the stomach.

Stop and consider that dog and cat teeth are not continually growing and being worn away because the crown is being continually eroded. A horse's teeth continually grow with the roots getting shallower every year. The problem is that teeth are not getting enough wear, a lot less than 60,000 grinding rotations daily. The head is not down long enough to stretch the dorsal spine, weakening the spine and adding to chiropractic problems.

With uneven wear of the teeth, occlusion problems occur, and, as humans who like things to be 'natural' we put feed bins at stable door height. This makes eating more difficult (compared with dogs and cats fed at floor level). When the head is at stable door height, the lower jaw drops back and there is no grinding of the upper first pre-molar on an opposite tooth, nor, in the case of the back of the last molar in the lower jaw.

After a time, there is a downward hook in the front of the upper jaw and an upward hook (ramp) at the back of the lower jaw. This leads to malfunction of the chewing mechanism; alters the amount of occlusion; reduces feed efficiency; and causes pain where the mandible meets the skull (the temporo-mandibular joint) which can lead to arthritis.

Now you put a bit in the animal's mouth and expect him to behave when your rein instructions cause pain. Bitting is another subject altogether, and is not covered here.

## Dentistry

Pre 1900, horse dentists took the above into account. In my days of doing horse dentistry (1959-2000), I just used to cut the aforementioned hooks and ramps and smooth them over with a rasp as well as clearing any sharp edges on the rest of the teeth. This has now been superseded by *whole of mouth dentistry* as practiced by accredited veterinary dentists and those certified by the College of Equine Dentistry of Australia (akin to that in the USA). At present there are insufficient individuals with such qualifications in Australia and New Zealand. The other group specialising in equine dentistry is the Veterinary Equine Dentists, and there is also an insufficient number of these. Speaking generally, veterinarians do not condone the work of lay dentists. This is an unfortunate state of affairs — especially for the welfare of the horse.

## Problems arising from a poor mouth

- Bit playing
- Lugging, hanging, head-throwing

- Bucking
- Avoiding being caught
- Back problems
- Lameness (emanating from neck area)

I would suggest you ask the horse dentist to show you what the mouth looks like before he starts work. For this, you will require a strong torch. Make sure he explains what needs to be done, and that he shows you the final result.

Horse owners, in general, are prepared to pay out for their horse's feet to be done every six to eight weeks. However they are less inclined to pay out to keep its teeth in good order. While this might well cost more initially, maintenance of good dentition costs a similar amount to shoeing. The advantage is that it would lead to a better controlled animal and reduce the risk of colic. In addition the cost of feed is very likely to be less because it would be used more efficiently.

**Note:**

- Feed at ground level.
- Pasture as much as possible.
- If no feed in pasture, give hay accordingly.
- Regular good dental care.
- Learn about bits. Most people use bits that are too small.

## ALIMENTARY PROBLEMS

### Colic

Panic! Panic! Panic! This is the general emotion encountered by horse owners. Calm down a minute. A horse is a panic merchant as well and will tell you it thinks it's dying. But what is colic? It's the same as in all species including humans – a tummy pain. Most colics are transitory and will right themselves, *but* don't take this for granted. By all means call your vet, but there are things you can do while waiting.

There are four main types of colic -

1. **Spasmodic (gaseous)** — Rolling, kicking
2. **Impaction** — Constipation, quiet, looks to side affected
3. **Twist** — Volvulus, full or partial
4. **Strangulation** — Intussusception

**Spasmodics** often correct themselves. However, in these cases you usually see the horse sweating, constantly getting up and down as well as rolling. Treatment advisable.

**Impactions** usually need treatment. These usually show in the form of discomfort, the horse looking around to the side where the impaction is. The horse may be either standing or down when doing this. Symptoms are similar when sand is present in the large gut.

**Twists** mostly require surgery. Here, there is usually excessive rolling and sweating and the gums turning slowly to dark red.

## Strangulation

> **Type 1**: Intussusception is when one piece of the gut telescopes into the other. Surgery essential.

> **Type 2**: When a loop of gut passes through a natural orifice, and the walls of the orifice prevent the blood supply reaching the gut loop which becomes gangrenous. Mostly surgical.

## Things you can do:

The common misconception, in my point of view, is 'walking the horse'.

If you have a stomach ache, do you want to walk about? No. You'd rather curl up with a hot water bottle on your stomach. So why walk the horse? To stop it rolling you say. Why stop it, I ask? In case it twists you say. Fallacy I say!

A horse will roll normally for pleasure. After exercise a horse will often roll. Its guts do not twist. In fact, a *treatment* for twist can be to roll the horse, sometimes under anaesthesia, with an arm in its rectum. So, *if* there is a twist, the horse is possibly trying to relieve it by rolling.

My suggestion is that you **keep the horse warm**.

I also suggest that you give it a bottle of warm flat beer.

Does this do any good? Many of my clients swear by it. But quite possibly the horse was going to get better anyway. At least it gives you something to do and makes you feel you are helping (which is why people walk their horses). Beer in humans certainly helps in gut cases and often 'keeps you regular'.

**Massaging** the (acupressure) points of the ears can also help.

**Another thing** you can do. Have someone hold the horse's head. Then take a towel and pass it under the horse to someone on the other side. You both take an end of the towel, and with it over the navel area, you both lift and hold for fifteen seconds. Relax for fifteen seconds and then repeat. This has the same effect as you rubbing your stomach. This I have found to be the most useful home treatment in the case of impaction or partial twist.

I have recently heard that **oranges** will help colic, particularly that caused during trail or endurance riding, though my personal experience of this is non-existent. This is an anecdote, and I am unsure why oranges would be helpful.

© 2015 R. H. Chapman

The ideas given above are not intended to replace veterinary treatment, but will give you something to do while waiting for the vet to arrive. This is helpful if your vet is many miles away or not available.

Most veterinary treatments are pain killers and antispasmodics, to alleviate symptoms while the horse improves on its own. Oils are given by your vet for impaction-type colic, and where dehydration from prolonged colic occurs, fluids are essential. But I must stress that this is a veterinary treatment.

In days of old, horsemen would dig a shallow trench, cast the horse and roll it on its back into the trench, then massage the abdomen with a plank for about 15-30 minutes before allowing the horse to get up.

## Recurrent Colics

These usually require veterinary advice. They can be caused as a result of worms (even after their elimination) or as a result of many other things including trauma and sand.

**A case history in point** — some years ago a horse called *Imgrime* went to Randwick from Canberra to race. It escaped the strapper and hit a four wheel drive in the car park. No apparent problem occurred and the horse was passed fit to race and raced okay.

About a week later it had what looked like a strangulated colic, *but* responded to an antispasmodic medication.

This colic occurred regularly over periods of 5 to 27 days. It responded to treatment each time until the eighth event, when it got progressively worse. Surgery was declined, so the horse was euthanised and an autopsy carried out. Apparently, the accident had caused a tear in the omentum (the curtain from which the intestines hang) through which a loop of gut had passed and become strangulated, causing peritonitis. One has to assume that the loop of gut had been going through this aperture each time. The antispasmodics relaxed the gut, so the loop fell out again. In the end, the loop must have travelled in too far and stayed there. The hole acted as a noose, stopping the blood supply to the strangulated loop of gut, which then became gangrenous, leading in turn to peritonitis.

## Brown Snake Bite

Brown snake bite I will cover later (under 'Other Conditions') but accurate diagnosis is needed before going to the expense of anti-venom. This usually presents as acute colic. The horse drops suddenly, then gets up, and suddenly drops again. This is ongoing, and pain killers have no impact.

**Diarrhoea**

This, in the horse, is one of the hardest things to clear up whether you are a layman or a veterinarian. From a vet's point of view, intravenous fluids are certainly necessary in acute cases, but when *not* acute there are a few things that seem to work.

Most horses with diarrhoea are **thirsty**. Give an alternate pail of water in which you have put **clay** and stirred. Also leave some clay in the stable/yard/paddock. Very often you will find the horse prefers the clay water or will chew the clay – this leaves a coating on the gut which soothes it. Even when a horse is not suffering from diarrhoea they will often dig to clay in their stables to eat it.

**Paspalum** is a jointed fibrous grass which when cut up as chaff and fed will often reduce the diarrhoea to 'slop' or even clear it up.

A **Vitamin A** supplement is useful as this aids repair of mucous membranes and thus has an affect on the gut lining, but is better in conjunction with other treatments.

**Probiotics** can be very helpful and these can be found in proprietary medications (ie Protexin).

An alternative is to replenish the **digestive microbes**. Take the faeces of a healthy horse and put them in a pail of water. Stir well and leave for an hour. Then strain it to get the worst of the solids out. Drench the horse with the remainder. What you are trying to do is replenish the correct digestive microbes. I prefer this latter to probiotics because the microbes in the gut are more specific to the horse and also its environment.

## Internal Parasites

Most horse owners regularly worm their horses, and of course your vet is the best person to advise you what to use and when to do so. We will talk about bots later in the ectoparasite section, so I won't repeat it here.

The tiny horse **tapeworm** has never, in my experience, caused a problem, but it is said that, in some areas where it is prevalent, it can be a cause of recurrent colic. This problem usually occurs at the junction of the small and large intestines and the blind gut (caecum).

The **bright red roundworm** known as *Strongylus vulgaris* has a life cycle where the larvae concentrate in the mesenteric artery. They create reactions, which narrow the size of the lumen (tunnel), and even cause some blood clotting. This in turn reduces the blood supply to the gut, so that when food reaches the affected area you get a 'cramping' of the gut muscle, causing colic. Also, for a similar reason, when you exercise the horse, more blood is needed to work the muscles, and therefore less is available to the gut, which of course is further lessened by the narrower vessels. Hence the horse gets colic.

Other large strongyles are not so detrimental and all are killed by the same worm treatment as are the small strongyles. This is not a text book on worm cycles so I am not going further into these.

I will, however, touch on two other types of worms that appear alarming to owners of horses.

The 'milk' worm or Parascaris looks like a 10-15 cm length of spaghetti. It is commonly seen in young animals, and less often in older horses. The life cycle is about 6 weeks and incorporates the liver. For this reason, I recommend at least fortnightly treatment for 4-6 treatments, but ask your vet.

Another worm is the pin worm which lay eggs around the anus and glues them there, causing gross itching as the glue dries and shrinks. This causes the horse to rub its tail region, often damaging skin around the buttocks. Part of the treatment is to wash the anus daily to clear the glue and eggs. Your vet will let you know the best treatments, but I usually treat every three weeks for at least four doses. The differential diagnosis for this, especially during the summer, is an allergy to gnat or small insect bites (sweet itch).

# COUGHS and COLDS

## Coughs

A **dry** cough is usually caused by a **herpes virus**, or dust in the environment. 'Live' dust, from hay etc, is worse than 'dead' dust like dirt. Most herpes viruses will clear in 10 - 21 days, but the horse should not be worked hard during this time. There is a vaccine against this which, although not one hundred percent effective, will allow you back to competition in 3 - 4 days, as this is usually the duration of the cough (vaccinated horses only).

A **moist** cough, with mucus production, is usually the sign of a **bacterial** infection and the attention of your vet is the best solution, especially if your horse is running a fever.

Following on from this, you must consider **strangles**, which is usually accompanied by swelling of the lymph nodes. This condition is not as serious in older horses as in the young. Vaccination has dubious value for strangles.

**NOTE:**

**Viral (herpes)** type coughs are **contagious** (pass through the air = airborne).

**Bacterial (strangles)** types are **infectious** (must come into 'contact' with the infection).

© 2015 R. H. Chapman

General advice is **NOT to work** your horses when they are coughing, as it could affect the heart.

**Chronic Obstructive Pulmonary Disease** (COPD) = broken wind/emphysema.

More common in ponies and horses stabled for long periods. It is the result of chronic infections and/or allergies to dust. In these cases, the lungs tear like you see in an old sponge. The lungs then hold matter because their elasticity is reduced, thus requiring coughing to remove it.

These horses are best left outside, and do keep fitter with exercise. They will cough at the start of exercise, but improve throughout work. Treatment is aimed at keeping the lungs clear. Your vet is the best person to advise you on your particular case.

## Colds

**Discharge or bleeding from one nostril** is usually sinus related: –
- By an infection left after a previous disease
- A cracked and infected tooth root
- A tumour
- An old fracture

These animals are best seen by your vet, who can use a scope, or x-ray, to see what is going on.

## Cough/Cold prevention

- Vaccination – Herpes/strangles/EI (equine influenza).

  Dampen feed, including hay. The best way is to place it in a net and saturate it. Leave it to drain for 8 - 12 hours before feeding.

- Feed at ground level.

- Leave in paddock, where there is less likelihood of picking up infections.

## EYES and EARS

### EYES

Stating the obvious, an animal has two eyes which are both delicate structures. The loss of one, therefore, is serious, the loss of *both* is disastrous. Although, one horse I found blind on a pre-purchase examination had been quite happy in its original habitat, but when moved to a different property exhibited the tentative behaviour of blindness.

Do not hesitate to contact your vet even if you consider the condition harmless. Without going into the complete anatomy of the eye I would like to comment on the pupil because this is a useful guide to your vet when you ring him/her.

> **Dilated pupil** – in our species the dilated pupil is always round, and when fully dilated leaves the iris as a narrow band surrounding the black-looking pupil. This occurs naturally in the dark, and as the surroundings get light, so the pupil constricts (gets smaller).

> **Constricted pupil** – in bright daylight the pupil is at its maximum constriction (smallest).

**Horses** need to see in front and sideways as much as possible. Hence the constricted pupil is **horizontal**. A point to remember in this case is that when you are riding your horse with its head collected and facing down, it can see very little distance ahead. Therefore, it has to have faith in its rider. Without that, you will have a horse with a tendency to play up because it will be trying to get its head up so that it can see where it is going.

## Weepy Eyes

Bilateral weepy eyes in horses are likely to be caused by an allergic response to flies, wind, dust, pollen, etc.

However, if only one eye is weepy and the eyeball appears clear, this can be an early sign of **uveitis**, especially if there is any constriction of the pupil in the dark.

This condition can be recurrent. Old names for this were ophthalmia or moon blindness — the latter name because of its likely repetitive occurrence.

Therefore, **call your vet** because this can become very serious and lead to the loss of the eye.

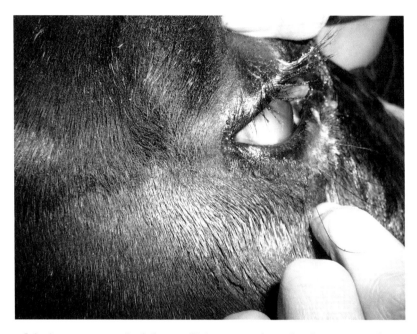

This is a very painful condition causing the horse to close its eye, often accompanied by a lot of tears. This is when at least the top layer of cells has been rubbed off the front of the eye. This should be treated as a matter of urgency by your vet before it gets deeper and maybe eventually rupture. Below are some treatments you can use until your vet shows up.

## Eye Preparations

Available, without prescription, from the pharmacy are Brolene eye drops or ointment, or Antistine Privine eye drops, which can help alleviate discomfort until the vet sees your animal. Antibiotic and atropine eye preparations are available from your veterinarian or on prescription from the pharmacy. All commercial eye drops/ointments are provided as sterile products but any unused portion is to be discarded after 28 days.

**On no account use preparations containing cortisone of any type** UNLESS prescribed by your veterinarian for the current condition. Do not use any left-over corticosteroid preparations.

Sometimes, particularly after extended antibiotic use, an ulcer can become infected by **fungus**. This is extremely serious and, therefore, if the ulcer being treated has not responded well and is mostly becoming more yellow and opaque, your vet will need to *see* the animal again and take a swab for microscopic examination.

A horse I was treating had this condition - confirmed by examination of a scraping from the lesion. Treatment was carried out three times daily with an anti-fungal agent into the eye and an anti- inflammatory medication by mouth, and it still took three months to come right. We had even considered removing the eye, but my client was a fighter so we persevered with treatment and the result was good — only a small scar remained.

**Under Eyes**

The nictitating membrane, or third eyelid, is well developed in reptiles and acts like the eyelids in

© 2015 R. H. Chapman

mammals. This is far less developed in the horse in which the most common lesion is cancer. Initial signs are just teary eyes. Most common in non-pigmented parts of the membrane.

The third eyelid is often used by your vet in operations when the corneal surface has been damaged. This will be stitched over the lesion.

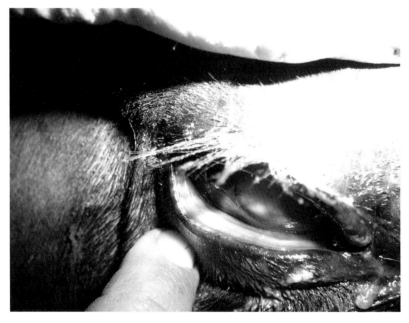

Another condition mostly seen on the lateral corner of the eye is a fleshy lump, which may or may not be a cancer but does seem to respond well to cortisone treatment by your vet.

Dark tumour type growths just outside the eyelids are

usually neurofibromas and appear to respond well to a BCG injection into the lesion by your vet.

## EARS

Ear conditions are not common in horses, the most common being ear mites. These mites cause head shaking, especially when the weather is hot or the horse is working and the ears get hotter. This causes the mites to become more active and move around hence irritation is more intense. Sometimes in these cases you will notice the hair on the leading edge of the ear to be much shorter or absent.

Treatment is easy. Just squirt **ivermectin** of any type into the ears at two weekly intervals for three treatments. I usually do not examine the ear first because this has to be done under heavy sedation or anaesthetic for the operator's safety.

### Foreign body

The most common of these are insects, especially flies. As you would expect this will drive a horse mad. However, this is usually self-limiting when the insect escapes. Less so if it dies! Then it does have to be removed. Don't try it! Leave it to your vet.

Any foreign body remaining in the ear will need to be

removed. This usually entails an anaesthetic so it's definitely a case for calling the vet.

Water, or fluids, in the ears have only a short effect so no treatment is necessary.

In general ear problems necessitate veterinary input.

# FOUNDER/LAMINITIS

### Founder (Laminitis)

Founder is basically an **ischaemia** (lack of blood) to the sensitive laminae — the network between the hoof wall and the pedal bone.

Symptoms are a desire to remain in one place. (It mostly affects the front feet: sometimes all four feet: very rarely the hind feet only). When the horse walks it tries to walk on its heels and hence has a rock-back action. This is particularly in the case of grass founder. There are three main types:

- **Grass founder** — mostly in ponies
- **Stress founder** — in race horses this is usually low grade or chronic. But if other horses gorge carbohydrates, and occasionally proteins, they generally become very sick.
- **Post-birth founder** — obviously mares only, it is associated with retention of part or all of the placenta (after-birth). Mare very sick to critical.

### Treatment

All founders need veterinary input but acute stress and post-birth founder can be *fatal* so don't waste time.

A client of mine had an older mare that had never foundered. In the Spring the mare was reluctant to move, and it was two weeks before my clients asked me to look at her. This turned out to be a medium grade grass founder which took six months to resolve, especially as infection and seedy-toe had followed.

# HORMONAL CONDITIONS

I do not intend to enter into any discussion on obstetrical hormonal dysfunction. This per se is a veterinary problem as it is usually complex!

Main hormonal problems seen in paddocked horses include :-

1. Swollen udder containing milk.

2. Stallion-like tendencies in geldings.

3. Cranky mares.

4. Mares behaving like stallions.

## Treatments of 1 to 4

1. The only treatment I know that may be effective, is to apply vinegar (preferably apple cider) to the udder three or four times daily. This condition is usually due to mares being on high oestrogen pastures.

2. Caused by the adrenal gland producing more testosterone than normal. Oestrogen is no good to counteract, but a long acting progesterone works well.

3. Probably oestrogenic. i.e. cystic ovaries. Likewise long acting or daily treatment progesterone works

well.

4.  Can be due to granulosa cell tumour of the ovary. Surgery only treatment.

**Conditions 2 to 4 require veterinary input.**

## Cushings Disease

Common in Horses 20 years or older. First sign is usually a long coat. Also a tendency to laminitis likely to be unresponsive to normal treatment routines. Very often these affected horses will live apparently comfortably for a long time.

Sometimes horses as young as 10 can have laminitic problems and this can be due to subclinical Cushings. Get your vet to check it out.

# MUSCULO-SKELETAL CONDITIONS

This perhaps is the hardest thing to describe and tell you what to do about it as diagnosis is the most important and most difficult part of it. I am going to include dentition in this section — and being most rostral (forward) will start with that.

## Dentition

In the old days we vets and lay dentists really only considered minor things like removing wolf teeth and rasping the points of the tongue side of the lower molars and premolars and the cheek side of the upper set. If the horse was parrot-mouthed, we watched for a downward spike (hook) of the first upper premolar (cheek) tooth and the upward spike of the last molar (cheek tooth) in the lower jaw (ramp). If the latter became too large it would dig into the upper jaw bone and the horse could not eat because it could not close its jaw effectively – this spike would then require cutting or grinding down to enable the jaw to resume natural function.

With an undershot jaw the reverse would be the case with the spike at the back of the upper jaw causing the same problem. The forward spikes cause some bridling problems.

Nowadays dentistry has become more of a speciality with

© 2015 R. H. Chapman

the use of power tools and new nomenclature. Some of the old dentists still only rasp teeth but the modern lay dentists have a diploma and often require vets to perform sedation on their patients. Many vets have also undertaken special training and of course can do their own sedation. Incisor teeth now play a great part and dentists are looking at bite and ease of lateral movement.

It has now been found that poor bite and chew can not only cause neck problems but also other problems down the spine. These problems are not necessarily only caused by eating, but also with riding patterns. Therefore proper dental care now becomes a 'MUST'.

Here is a story against myself, which I tell so others do not make the same error:

57 years ago in England, vets seldom used a gag (speculum) but just pulled the tongue to one side to do the rasping. In this particular case the horse eventually became so emaciated — with no specific cause isolated by myself or any other vet — that the animal was euthanised.

Post mortem NOTHING was found until, exasperated, I opened the head to find two ramps from the lower jaw had embedded SO deeply into the upper jaw that the horse could not grind its teeth together. It was literally starving.

**LESSON**: ALWAYS use a gag (speculum)

## Lameness

Lameness is one of the hardest things to describe, which is difficult because correct diagnosis is very important.

Lameness is a musculo-skeletal condition. Some causes are obvious and others hidden. Some are probably not called lameness because, while the gait is still okay, the animal responds poorly to riding. Most horses over eight years of age have some degeneration of many joints — the most being noticeable in the hocks.

Gait is often altered imperceptibly. Therefore, most performance horses over eight years old are on a joint treatment. Many race horses start this treatment as prevention.

## Arthritis

Arthritis is common post trauma. Often there is also low grade degeneration gradually turning into more loss of cartilage and bony invasion. It is only obvious if the joint gets knobbly. This is seen in knees and hocks mainly, but may also be seen in the fetlock joints and below.

There are some good treatments these days and this is the time to discuss things with your vet.

# MORE MUSCULO-SKELETAL CONDITIONS

## Tendons

If these are swollen or enlarged — and mostly you'll only notice the flexor tendons (superficial and deep) where there is *no* lameness — you can try cold/ice treatment. Treatments such as a methylated spirit and ice bandage, such as **Penetrene** or **Dencorub** etc. can be tried. If there is any lameness, the tendon itself may well be damaged, so once again a veterinary problem. Please note that if things don't clear up quickly, call your vet to get a proper diagnosis before you do irreparable damage.

## Bog Spavin

This is hock swelling — below inside, above outside. Pushing on the swelling will cause the other side to bubble. The usual cause is conformation — straight hock. It is not normally treated but, on occasions rubbing in castor oil has worked. Note, it is a mild blister, so after about three days the horse will resent this. Stop immediately. Repeat two weeks later. If no improvement, cease treatment. If it does appear to work, keep repeating. Vet treatment will be required if lameness is concurrent. However, little can be done to correct the swollen aspect of the hock to look normal.

## Saddle

How do you tell if a saddle is the problem — especially if it has been fitted? Mostly you'll find the long muscles running down the under side of the neck are painful. Sometimes putting pressure with your fingers to the side of the withers will also prove painful. If the back is sore it is more obvious. High-withered horses often have problems with the saddle. In these cases, a piece of carpet under-felt cut and sloping from beneath the withers to behind the withers will raise the saddle from the withers.

I had one case of an endurance horse that *always* played up going down a steep slope. Obviously the saddle came down on the withers. This simply needed a crupper to solve the problem. To ease the neck muscle problem, I use a Penetrene/vinegar preparation; just wiped on before exercise.

If you have a wither that is sore on one side, there is a certain amount of embarrassment for a vet having to suggest that the rider is either right or left 'arsed' — in other words, a tendency to push the saddle in, on one side. It happens often, so if this appears your horse's affliction, look to yourself first!

## Neck

As mentioned previously, neck pains can be caused by saddle fit, but this is muscular. However, neck (bone) injuries or slight misalignments can be caused by falls, or by pulling back on ropes or halters during breaking or at any later time. This usually shapes up as stiffness — particularly to one side — or sometimes as a shortened gait. This often requires chiropractic treatment, with or without an anaesthetic, according to severity, the horse's temperament and the lesion concerned.

## Bursitis

This is not often diagnosed and is more common than we suspect, mostly diagnosed by a veterinary surgeon. The only ones I have come across are shoulder bursae and those near the hip on what we call the trochanter. I believe these are usually due to trauma and require veterinary treatment.

## Hamstrings and Haunches

I suspect trauma is the usual cause of problems — being kicked by another horse probably the commonest. Seen by pain down the back of the leg — mainly between the pin bone and the back of the stifle. Occasionally the muscle appears string-like — that is no elasticity — and the gait shown is a sudden snatch-back as the hind leg can only go so far forward before the 'string' stops it.

I have twice seen this condition bilaterally and do not know its cause. There is no treatment that I know, other than surgery (which is mostly successful). Maybe massage and/or physiotherapy would help.

## Capped Elbow - Capped Hock

Swelling often painful over point of hock and point of elbow — veterinary advice and treatment recommended. Ice can be used as first aid. Ichthammol/Phlegmon may also be applied. in the early stage. Your vet may drain these and inject cortisone. Bandaging the site is pretty well impossible!

## Tying Up

More common in mares. Horses generally have to be on hard feed to get this condition which is exemplified by stiffness, and hard loin and rump muscles. Will definitely occur if the horse is fed concentrates before exercise; and in this case will be acute.

This is a milder form of **azoturia**, which is a condition commonly seen in English Hunters during a hunt. They seize up, and if ridden, not floated home, they often die

© 2015 R. H. Chapman

or become long-term invalids. One symptom of bad tying up, or azoturia, is a ruby red or dark coffee coloured urine and this denotes a breakdown of myoglobin in the muscles.

For example, one owner gave his endurance horse a large oat feed both the night before and the morning of an endurance ride. The horse went for three kilometres before it needed to be floated back to base and then home, so bad was the condition.

Treatment is veterinary.

Prevention, or treatment in mild cases :-

- **Willow leaves.**

- **Aspirin:** a minimum of 20 to 50 x 300mg tablets daily for a minimum of four days. Dose up to 25 grams daily is okay.

- Feed **pipe clay** or potters clay as a substitute (this I consider the best therapy of any)

- Sometimes **trace minerals** will work, especially selenium with vitamin E.

An anecdote regarding pipe clay comes from a certain hill in the Crimea. The hill was known to consist of pipe clay. After hard riding, when the cavalry horses were unsaddled, they'd all go over and get stuck into the clay. Next day they were all refreshed and eager to go.

Afterwards, pipe clay was used regularly as a treatment and prevention.

I have used it successfully in treatment and also as prevention with excellent results. The only problem is finding it. Hence, I suggest potters clay as a substitute. In recent times I have found colloidal trace elements to be of benefit.

## Sore Back

Two unusual treatments for sore backs. Homeopathic treatment will be under that section.

1. Hang an **infra-red lamp** over the sore area which you have previously smeared with oil. The lamp needs to be two to three feet above the area, and the treatment is applied for about 30 minutes.

2. I have tried the following with great success especially with a Waler stallion suffering with a sore back. Its back was very sore four days before a 160km endurance ride. The stallion completed the ride in time!

   Take the skin from a freshly killed sheep, lay the skin over the back, flesh side down and tie in place. In summer this can get very smelly and maggoty. There is no scientific basis for this, so it's an old wives tale that works. It's worked well for me on more than one occasion!

## Massage

This is a specialised area and trained professionals are well qualified to do muscle and physiotherapy work. Most of their work, I suspect, complements veterinary and chiropractic treatment.

A specialised, very gentle form of massage is known as the **Tellington-Jones** technique which is a special course on its own. This can also be of use especially where relaxation is needed.

## RESTRAINTS

When restraining horses it is advisable for the handler NOT to wear rings or bracelets. I have seen a finger torn off when a ring has got entangled with the lead, and also a badly broken and torn wrist in the case of the handler wearing a bracelet.

**Twitch** – this is the commonest used but not my first choice. A twitch is a loop rope/string attached to a short or long handle or ring.

It is looped over the horse's nose and twisted tight. Besides being uncomfortable, this action is believed to release endorphins that reduce pain and calm the horse.

If the horse is not too strong a twitch can be put on by placing the loop round your knuckles, grabbing the horse's nose and, with the other hand, putting the loop over the horse's nose, and then twisting.

Otherwise, you can hold the horse over the bridge of the nose while you grasp the nose with the other hand. Get someone else to twist the rope (using of course the ring or handle).

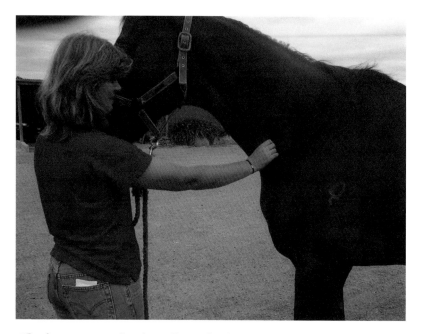

**Christmas grip (neck twitch)** – This in my opinion is the first choice provided it works on the particular animal being handled.

All you do is grab a large hunk of skin in the centre of where the neck joins the shoulder.

Hold hard — after a while your hand tires and it is difficult to straighten your fingers. If the horse is very tense, so is the skin which means it may be difficult to grab.

In this case, turn the horse's head towards you. This will loosen the skin that side and enable you to grab hold of a chunk.

This grip is particularly useful when a horse keeps throwing up its head when you are trying to treat the eyes or doing an intravenous injection.

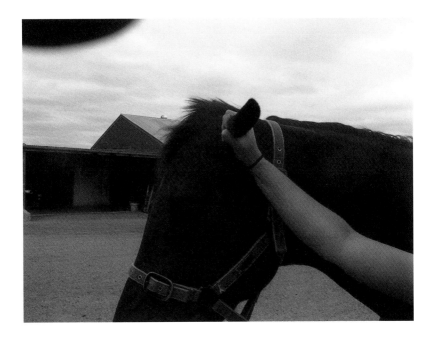

**Ear grab** – I call this an ear grab not a twitch. An ear twitch is when you grab the ear and screw it.

An alternative to this is to put a twitch loop over the ear and screw it up.

I believe just grabbing the ear and holding it tight with your weight on it is quite sufficient and has far less likelihood of making a horse head shy or ear shy as it

© 2015 R. H. Chapman

does not hurt, but just has him off balance.

BUT Remember the hyoid bones (swallowing apparatus) can be broken if too much vigorous pulling down on the ears. Also if too much pull pressure is put on the tongue.

**Poll hold** - hold both ears with one hand which is placed on the horse's poll — useful if you are a tall person.

**Blindfold** – one or both eyes. By covering one eye only, the horse tends not to panic. It is somewhat disorientated and is therefore more concerned with getting orientated than with what you are trying to do to it. The double blindfold is generally used to get a horse to go where it does not want to go.

Having blindfolded the horse, you turn it around three or four times so it loses direction. Then you lead it to where you want it to go.

This is best done with a towel so that, if the horse panics, the blindfold can be quickly pulled off to prevent the horse from galloping off blind. Pacifiers and blinkers can also be used, but do not block out both eyes.

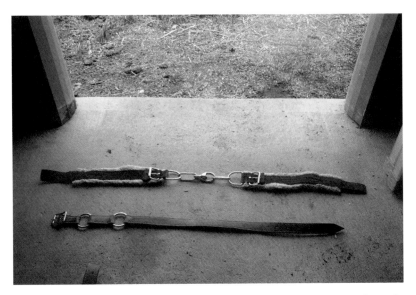

**Knee hobbles (straps)** – These are straps around each knee joined together by another strap. This reduces the ability for a horse to strike (front leg kick) and, of course, limits its movement.

This is not one of my favourite forms. I prefer the next method.

**Foot halter** – This is a leather loop joined to another leather loop by a length of rope (length dependent on size of horse).

One loop is placed around the fore fetlock and the other on the hind fetlock of the same side — you can use one on each side — but one side is usually sufficient.

© 2015 R. H. Chapman

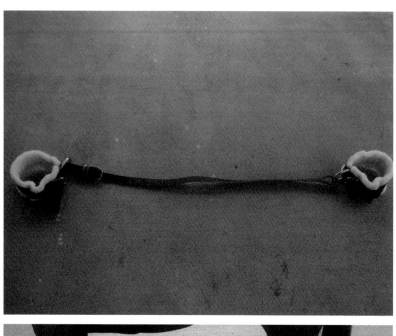

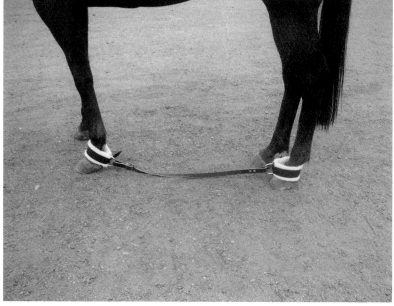

Here, if a horse tries to kick it pulls its *own* front leg back, and if it tries to strike it is held back by its back leg – very effective.

**Tips**

Just a few handling tips.

If trying to raise a foreleg to look at the foot: -

- Pull back on the chestnut — the reflex is to lift the leg.
- Squeeze forward of the flexor tendons behind the cannon.
- If there are hairs (feathers) on the back of the fetlock, you can pull on these.

If trying to raise the hind leg:

- as for 2 and 3 above
- or just pull forward on the flexor tendons.

© 2015 R. H. Chapman

# SKIN PROBLEMS

**Warts** - juvenile warts – **papillomatosis** is caused by a virus, and generally cover the muzzle, face and round the eyes. These will self eliminate in six to twelve weeks. Warts can appear in older horses — and can be removed surgically — but the majority of these 'warts' are not warts but sarcoids.

In the late 1950s, a colleague of mine in Devon, England, went to a farm where several young cattle were covered in warts. He told the farmer to wait ten weeks and the warts would disappear. In exactly ten weeks, they disappeared. And he got the reputation that he could remove warts by casting a spell over an animal!

This ten-week pattern is the same in young horses.

## Sarcoids

There are three types:

1.  **Cutaneous** — look like rough skin
2.  **Warty growths**
3.  **Pedunculated** — a big warty growth, connected to the body by a thin neck, usually on the limbs

**Treatments**

- Surgical removal
- Cryosurgery
- Combination of the above
- Chemotherapy
- Emu oil - 20mL daily for 5 - 6 weeks – non scientific.

One of my clients had a horse with a sarcoid on the commissure of the lips, which was surgically removed twice, by another veterinarian. Other lesions on the cheek and under the eye were also removed. When these procedures were unsuccessful, I was contacted, and tried cryosurgery twice, clearing all but the lesion on the lips.

I heard from the client some six months later, indicating that she had given 20ml of emu oil orally at exactly 5pm daily for five weeks. Photographs showed no evidence of the lesion on the lips and, at the time of writing, some six years later, there has been no recurrence. Unfortunately I have lost the photographic evidence.

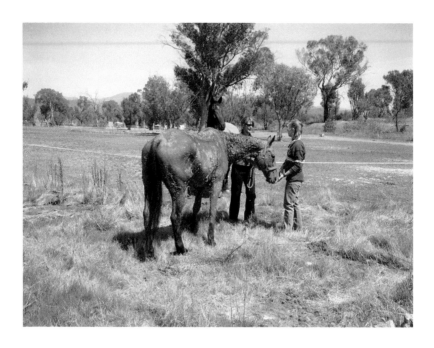

## Sarcoidosis

It is very difficult to treat and seldom diagnosed until advanced. There is gradual loss of virtually all hair, and there is also itchiness, with the horse getting cranky. Sarcoid-like cutaneous lesions occur throughout the body organs. It is very rare and mostly fatal, the horse being virtually bald in the end.

**Queensland Itch or Sweet Itch** - these are both allergies to insect bites. Queensland itch is basically on the head, neck and withers and is mostly found in tropical areas: whereas Sweet Itch is round the tail and rump in cooler climes. The latter is often mistaken for worms as the horse is seen rubbing its tail whenever possible. Treatment is with antiallergenic preparations and insecticidal washes or anti-fly sprays. A light rug is a reasonable prevention item as it reduces the area that insects can bite.

## Greasy Heel

This is caused by photosensitivity and moisture allowing the *Dermatophilus* in the skin to multiply and cause a painful condition of the skin layers. The white portions of the leg are commonest areas for greasy heel as these are more susceptible to sunlight, and if the horse is on a high red clover diet, the white portions become even more sensitive.

The lesions normally produce exudative scabs, under which the *Dermatophilus* flourishes. However, removal of these hard scabs can increase problems by damaging underlying skin more, and thus allowing the infection to grow deeper. Only parenteral antibiotics will get to the lesions unless topical treatment is combined with DMSO. *Dermatophilus* is an anaerobic (no oxygen) infection which likes carbon dioxide and also flourishes on moisture.

## Prevention

An easy way is to cover white areas of the legs with motor

oil - not sump oil. Honey, grease, oils will do if painted on with a brush daily. Unfortunately, too few people bother to do this and do not worry until the condition occurs.

Prevention can only happen if moisture is kept from the skin, which improves if the white portions are darkened.

A greasy, coloured zinc cream is fine also.

**Treatment**

Whatever you do, **don't** wash with water.

- You can experiment with your own mixture of grease, oil, honey or fat (like lard) with an antimicrobial such as sulphur, tea tree oil, copper sulphate, antimicrobial powder, or benzimadols - Panacur/Benzelmin. Charcoal can also be added to make a dark dressing.

- If you must remove a scab, honey or honey with yoghurt are effective. Hydrogen peroxide 1% or 2% also softens scabs, but the disadvantage is that it forms oxygen and water. Washing soda can also be used but also has the disadvantage of water. These all have to be bandaged for about 1 - 2 hours although honey (organic) can be left on indefinitely.

- Treatment should extend about 10cm above and below the apparent limit of the lesion.

- If water must be used, make sure you use something oily as a base afterwards.

- I have made my own ointment for persistent cases with sunscreen base plus a silver ointment or other fungicide plus a cortisone, cloxacillin and occasionally nystatin. This I have found best following the yoghurt and honey to get rid of the scabs.

## Ringworm

There are two types: -

- **Microsporum** - small lesions

- **Trichophyton**

Besides treating the animal, you must treat rugs and also spray tack and stable walls and door. Diagnosis of the animal is done by your vet.

Treatments can include iodine preparations. The benzimadols drugs, as with greasy heel, and commercial anti-fungal washes or ointments which are available from your vet.

## Ectoparasites

Parasites that live under or on the skin. In Australia the following are the main ectoparasites (outside the body) you are likely to come across.

- Ear mites
- Leg mites
- Harvest mites
- Ticks
- Biting insects – gnats, flies
- Lice
- Bots

**Ear mites** — as named these are located in the ear. They become more active and cause more itching as the environment heats up. Hence they appear worse in summer and also when the horse is worked, being one of the causes of head shaking. Full examination of the internal ear canal will require a heavy sedative or anaesthetic prior to examination. Mites can be seen with an otoscope. Other than this, the leading edge of the ear may well have no hair or at least a thinning edge.

**Treatment:** Before such an examination (and to save money) it may well be worth putting *ivermectin* (using a sheep drench) into the ear. This will kill the mites: it should be repeated in three weeks to ensure eggs and larvae do not produce mature mites and so allow the infection to continue.

**Leg mites** — seen mostly in the feathers of draft horses

such as Shires and Clydesdales. Symptoms are itching and stamping of the feet and also some noticeable inflammation at skin level with possibly a crusty excretion, not to be confused with canker, which is a moist gooey type of excretion.

Treatment: Once again, oral and local *ivermectin* is the best treatment.

**Harvest mites** — these mites are found, as you would expect, where grasses are mature. They seldom cause trouble but in some instances spark greasy heel. I sometimes therefore, incorporate ivermectin in my treatment of greasy heel.

**Ticks** — uncommon south of mid-NSW. In Australia they are endemic in many areas of Queensland and north NSW.

Treatment is to spray the whole animal.

**Lice** — there are two types, sucking and biting. These are both normally seen in the head/neck/wither and back. Usually during mid to late winter and horses are usually not very thrifty (strong and healthy). Is this due to the lice? Or do lice infect unthrifty horses? This is back to the chicken versus the egg argument!

Lice lay eggs known as 'nits' which hatch to larvae and progress to adult.

Treatment should be followed up in three weeks. There

are many proprietary lice treatments mostly washes. *Ivermectin* can be used as a pour on and also works especially with sucking lice, when used as a drench.

**Bots** – the fly is not strictly an ectoparasite, but when laying its eggs on the horses legs, shoulders, neck etc, they cause the horse to get irritable and often to gallop about. Hence it is known as the 'gad fly'. Bots will be dealt with in the internal parasite section.

**Biting insects** - gnats, midges, horse (biting) flies. These are not strictly parasites, but can, and often do, cause allergic skin problems which, when a horse has been sensitised, can cause a widespread reaction from only one or two bites. These take the form of body, and especially neck, lesions with loss of hair, known as Queensland itch, though of course not isolated to Queensland.

A milder form known as sweet itch occurs over the base of the tail and causes irritation which is often confused with pin or whip worms.

**Prevention**

To prevent 'biting' taking place the usual procedure is to use a light blanket and spray the exposed parts with a repellent.

However, recently available are plaques that can be

plaited into the mane and tail, which will give repellent action for weeks. I can see these becoming more efficient in the near future.

Some disadvantages are that, if these plaques are removed, (such as for shows, etc) for more than half an hour, they take 3 days to be effective again.

Maybe placing them on another horse for that short time would alleviate this problem. In any of the above cases, the severity of the condition will make you decide whether to call your vet or not.

## Alopecia (Balding)

Commonly one finds in late summer and late winter, horses seem to lose hair around the face, ears and neck in particular. I used to think this was fungal or parasitic, but samples taken were always negative.

Funnily, these animals cleared up in spring or in autumn as the case may be.

My feeling was that this cleared up because of the treatment of one of my two favourite vets — Dr Green. Grass provides things such as vitamin A when it is particularly succulent. This is stored in the liver. I have felt that these stores run low at the end of summer and winter.

Hence my treatment for this is a highly concentrated

Vitamin A supplement.

Sadly these come and go. Duphusaol Plus and Crown have come and gone. Now I use Olivitasol. These are oral preparations, injectable ones are available but are in an oily base and can irritate the horse, so should not be injected in large doses in one site.

Of course, cod liver oil is still available!

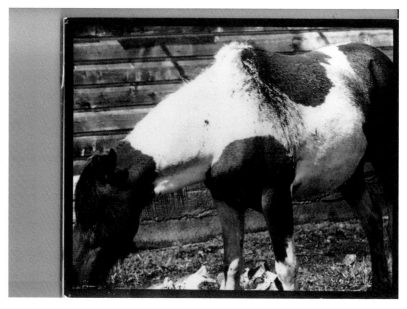

## Poll Evil and Fistulous Withers

These are abscesses like breakouts at the poll or withers, the latter to be differentiated from other forms of sore or infected withers. The cause is mostly a germ called *Brucella* and was often caused by contact with cattle.

However, Brucellosis (contagious abortion) has now been eradicated (in Australia) so this condition is rarely seen. Brucellosis is a zootic disease: that is, it can be transferred to humans.

As an anecdote — my personal second attack of Brucellosis in 1979 was from a horse with fistulous withers which I refused to touch. But, unfortunately, I had touched the wood of the yard where the horse was contained. I then spent over a week in hospital with a meningitic brucellosis from which I was lucky to pull through. My first attack was from aborting cattle.

Although I was using gloves while calving or removing retained afterbirth to prevent skin contact infection, the mode of entry was through inhalation which at the time was not recognised, and could have been prevented by dampening down the rear end of the cow.

**A condition which can be confused with fistulous withers** is a very painful condition on the wither usually initiated by the rug.

This generally presents as a weeping sore like an ulcer. It can be very resistant to treatment even with antibiotics or cortisones both topically or parenterally.

I find **hypericum cream** which also contains **calendula** is very good for these, but veterinary opinion may well be sceptical about this.

## Hooves

Finally in the skin section, I'm going to include the hoof of the horse.

In nature, horses in summer continually walk into rivers to cool their feet, but they do this less in winter. The hoof needs a certain amount of water, but in domestication it is not always available. Hooves and soles tend to get hard in summer, and softer in winter with the soles sometimes becoming soggy, with a tendency to get infected.

Topical hoof treatment is sometimes necessary — in summer to keep the water in; and in the winter to keep it out. Several are sold on the market but often change.

An old, well-tried product is **Stockholm tar.**

## Hoof Tonics (Oral)

Looking to hoof quality, apart from the water factor, we are looking for constituents that improve the horn. Ask your farrier.

- **Biotin** has been proven scientifically to improve foot quality, but is expensive.

- When I have put a horse on a supplement called **Equilibrium**, I have had farriers remark on the hoof improvement and to ask owners what they are doing differently.

- There is also a **colloidal mineral** preparation for horses which appears to help.

## Melanoma — Neurofibroma

These look alike and are easily muddled in horses. They are common to all species but probably most malignant in the pig.

In horses melanoma is commonly diagnosed round the eyelids, anus and lower side of the tail. They are most commonly found in greys. Most of these 'melanomas' are actually neurofibromas.

However, the treatment, if it is going to be done, is usually surgical or cryosurgical.

## Neurofibroma

Tumours on the eyelids are the ones that need most care in treatment because it is very easy to alter the lid margins and cause eye problems. I have found that injecting into these tumours with **human BCG vaccine** to be the most satisfactory. Chemotherapy with **cisplatin** will also be effective.

Dr. Richard H Chapman B.V.Sc.

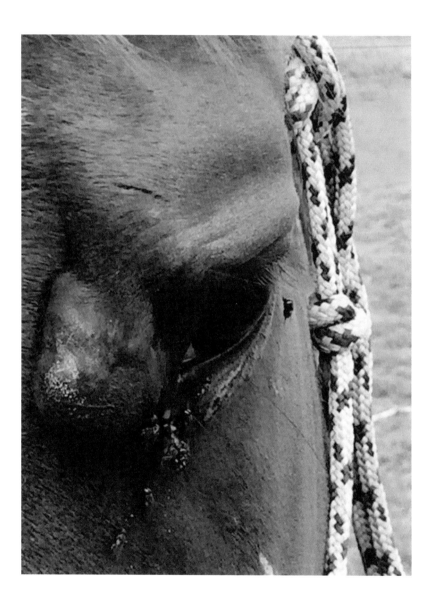

Tumours round the tail and anus are not problematical

until they involve the anal sphincter, so treatment is preferable before this occurs.

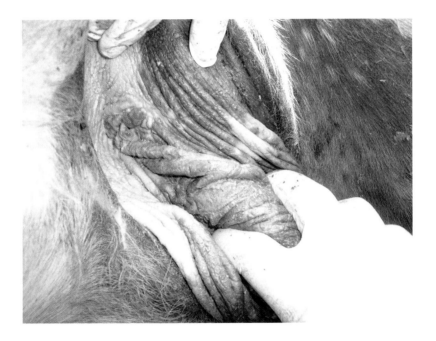

# WOUNDS

Treatment of wounds is very much up to the individual and that includes veterinarians. I am, therefore, not going into a lot of detail on every aspect of wound healing and treatment, but just give a few tips to try and reduce costs and prolongation of treatment.

## Burns

Treatment is of course related to severity. Some require euthanasia and most need veterinary care. However, as an initial treatment I use cold water (if early), and mixtures containing organic (untreated) honey. This includes a honey mix with such things as Unvita cream (vitamin A), yoghurt (natural, preferably home made) or anything that is solar protective.

## Cuts and Abrasions

Cold hose first if you can.

Many of these of course need suturing. Those lesions in the lower limbs of horses do not often respond well to stitching due to the tightness of the skin, and suturing these is basically to give a 'skin bandage'. What I am telling you now, can be done as a first aid measure whilst considering calling a vet, or waiting for their arrival, or getting smaller animals to the clinic.

To staunch bleeding, apply as many spider webs as you

can find over the wound, and then pressure bandage if that is possible (this cannot be done on the body or high up on the limbs). The bandage should start above or below the wound, whichever way is best to push the skin over the lesion. On the body, you seldom find a wound that causes severe bleeding so in these cases you can usually await treatment by a vet.

The old remedy was to throw a handful of lime over the wound and let the animal get on with it!

**Wounds near the eye** should be seen by a vet — most especially those affecting the eyelid margins. Any damage in that area may well cause some dysfunction of the lid. One of two things usually results.

If the lid dysfunction leaves part of the eye uncovered when blinking, the eye may dry out and chronic ulcers may form. Alternatively, the eyelid may turn in slightly, causing the eyelashes to irritate the surface of the eyeball.

An anecdote about the spider's web occurred when I did a ligature removal of a wart on the eyelid of a friend. Did it bleed?! He then told me he was on warfarin anti-clotting treatment. So we grabbed a few cobwebs and applied them to his eye. Repeated 4 hours later and no drama at all! Supposedly cobwebs contain antibacterials so no infection either.

## Proud Flesh (Hypergranulation)

In horses, an open bare wound on leg extremities, is very

prone to proud flesh. A great stimulant for this is water.

I realise that initially we cold hose a wound, and I also realise that when a bandage is removed the wound is 'yucky' and smelly and we feel we need to wash it. No problem.

But when finished hosing, RINSE WITH SALINE, preferably normal saline. If you are making this up at home, I suggest you boil up a litre of water with a half tablespoon/one tablespoon of salt. This will negate the effect of any water remaining on the wound and reduce proud flesh formation.

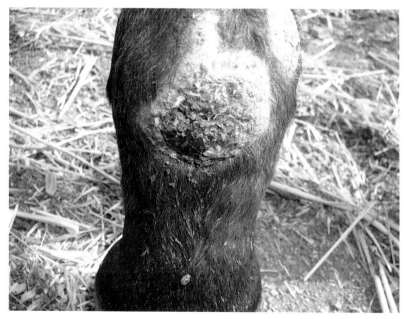

**Bandaging Wounds of the forelimb.**

I suggest these be bandaged in the normal way but not daily after the first few days.

I put on a firm bandage and leave it on as long as possible — 7 to 10 days. Let the wound 'stew' in its own juices. When you take the bandage off—BOY does it smell!! You can then hose it, but, finish with saline, dry, and redress.

A little trick to reduce the smell is to leave some of the dressing cotton wool poking out top and bottom, then, daily pour some bleach diluted to 2% onto the cotton wool at the top of the dressing. By leaving the dressing on for this length of time speeds up the healing and saves a lot of money!!

As a footnote, humans with bad abrasions, such as motorcycle accidents are treated in this way, with often a fibreglass cast over the top!

**Applications to reduce or negate the formation of proud flesh are**:

- **Insulin** — a prescription drug and therefore only used under the auspices of a veterinary surgeon.

- **Zinc sulphate** — As a powder from the chemist. If mixed with castor oil tends to be irritant, so use straight or better still in conjunction with Yellow

Lotion.

- **Yellow Lotion**
- **Pressure bandage**
- **Anti-proud flesh application** — zinc oxide, lead sub-acetate, *Dicks Solution*
- **Copper sulphate** — Used more for cutting back proud flesh – do not use *under* bandage. The powder can be ground into proud flesh and will cut it back over 24 hours. It does tend to leave a bigger scar but is useful especially when proud flesh is sliced off as it helps stem bleeding. Silver nitrate is used for humans but is more expensive than copper sulphate.
- **Prednoderm or Dermapred** — These are commonly used. They contain cortisone which reduces proud flesh but also tends to retard the rate of healing. Use of this is according to personal preference.
- **Lotagen or Healogen** — This is a very good product and is available as a lotion or a cream. I prefer the lotion as you can use this concentrated or diluted to suit your needs.
- **DMSO** — dimethylsulphoxide
- **Maggots** — If these get into the wound they help

debride the rotten flesh. They can stay a while but *not* long enough to eat healthy tissue — get rid of them then. Copper sulphate solution or DMSO works well!

## Bandaging Wounds of the Lower Limbs

After the first two to three days, the longer the bandage can be left on, all the better. Let the wound 'stew in its own juices'. Boy does it smell when you take the bandage off!

You can help this and the wound if you leave a little cotton wool protruding above and below the bandage, and pour daily about 100ml of 2% bleach on the cotton wool at the top of the bandage.

Dressings can be left on for seven to ten days. Results are amazing and cost a lot less than daily dressings, and the regenerating skin is left undisturbed.

## Puncture Wounds

These are another thing altogether. Puncture wounds entering a joint, in any animal, require veterinary attention so I'll go no further with that now.

These may be identified by seeing a straw coloured fluid coming out of the wound.

Other puncture wounds whether they be bites, wire

punctures, or anything else, require the same type of treatment by a vet — with the exception of the horse's foot which we will tackle later.

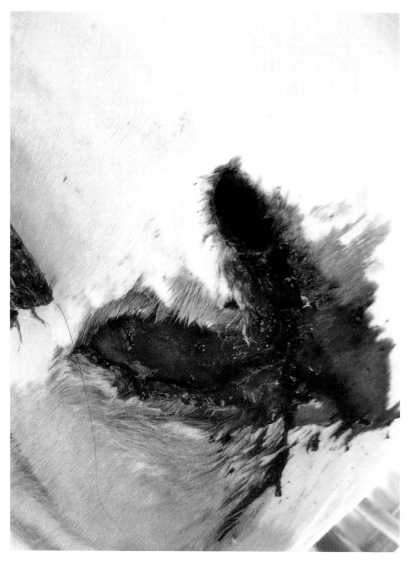

*Any* puncture wound is like an injection - an injection of infection. A poultice or drawing ointment such as **icthyol (ichthammol) or Magnoplasma** is useful BUT NOT ENOUGH. In dogs and cats, untreated puncture wounds invariably lead to abscess formation, which then bursts or needs lancing. In the horse, puncture wounds sometimes lead to abscesses. In the muscle, which is common, they lead to a nasty infection often proceeding to tetanus, unless immunised, or a necrotic type lesion.

Therefore, all puncture wounds need to be aggressively attacked with antibiotics and hence veterinary help is essential. ESSENTIAL.

That is, **ALL puncture wounds require veterinary attention** — if left too late the treatment will be longer, and may need some form of surgery, and will be much more expensive. If the puncture wound leaves a large draining wound, such as the removal of a large piece of wood low down in the belly muscle, lavage may well be sufficient!

A homeopathic treatment for punctures is Ledum pal 30C (3 times a day for 3 days).

Before dealing with the foot I would like to tell you now the sequel of the body reaction to TRAUMA – wounds –

tissue damage.

ANY TRAUMA to tissue, especially the horse, causes a release of prostaglandin which causes swelling and pain. The swelling allows the tissue to supply a good medium for bacteria to infect.

Therefore the first line of treatment is ANTI-PROSTAGLANDIN **not** Penicillin or other antibiotics as is the common belief.

Infection is noted by heat – redness – and pain at the slightest touch – not associated with the pain of touching a wound.

Non-steroidal anti-inflammatory drugs such as phenylbutazone or copper indomethacin (cualgesic) are ANTI-PROSTAGLANDIN – and if given soon after injury are probably all that is necessary with the exception of the puncture wound. The old bush treatment was kerosene and lime — and used to be quite effective!

## Hoof Problems

I would advise veterinary attention to any injuries of the coronary band. These injuries, even with treatment, will mostly cause some problem with hoof growth and quality, so the more the damage can be limited, the better the outcome. The resulting damage to the horn of the hoof and its growth will need constant farrier care, and often requires veterinary/farrier co-operation.

Damage to the wall of the hoof, as when a shoe is pulled off, can usually be treated by a good farrier — so unless the damage is severe this is probably your first point of call. However, if damage is excessive it would be wise to call your vet.

## Puncture Wounds of the Foot

The worst of these is a deep puncture in the frog. It is difficult to open and drain and may go into the navicular bursa. **Definitely a vet situation** even if it seems OK at the start. Many of these — if veterinary treatment is delayed — will lead to euthanasia! Other areas can penetrate the pedal (coffin) bone causing osteomyelitis and expensive treatment.

Virtually all puncture wounds will lead to abscess formation if not treated straight away.

## First Aid

This is what you can do to reduce problems. Remember: a nail in the foot is an injection of infection. Don't just pull out a nail if you find one — regardless of where in the foot. First clean the foot well — just water is okay. Float kerosene or iodine on the foot specifically over the nail or penetrating object then slowly pull the nail out —

wiggle it – stop 2 or 3 times during the process. This allows the fluid to penetrate the hole as it slides down the shaft of the nail.

Once the foreign object is out, either cut a hole right down to blood or just cut a circular mark and call your vet who will know what to do. The old bush people didn't have vets handy and this treatment alone was often all that was needed.

There is NO POINT putting a poultice on the foot unless there is a large enough hole to let the infection be pulled out. If antibiotics and/or a drain hole are not used, then these eventually proceed to abscessation plus or minus something more serous depending on the area of puncture as stated previously.

## Foot Abscess

Treatment for this is all the same, in principle, with veterinarians often having their own specific way. I'll just tell you mine.

If there is a puncture and I know where it is, I will cut a large hole in the sole or frog until I reach the underlying tissues. If pus emerges, and this is usually dark grey or black, I will apply a poultice or something like ichthammol (Phlegmon) and put the animal on antibiotics.

If I can't find a puncture or obvious pain point, I do not cut the sole in search of finding this. This is because over my time I have found that farriers have found it difficult to shoe the horse later — they call us vets FEET BORERS! Anyway, sometimes after doing all of this it may be the result of a seedy toe infection — not always starting at the sole — where you can see it and follow it up until it heads into the sensitive laminae.

These conditions I often leave, or suggest the whole foot including coronary band be poulticed. However lame the horse is, I do not use antibiotics at this stage as the horse will improve for a while — the abscess doesn't burst — and as soon as you leave off the antibiotics, the pain recurs.

Eventually the infection will burst at the coronary band. That is the time for antibiotics and also to see if you can find a lesion in the sole or white line directly beneath the breakout. After a course of antibiotics, healing is usually complete.

However, you may find a fault, where the abscess burst, that grows down the hoof over the next 12 months. Watch, and get your farrier to watch the white line at each shoeing, because a seedy toe-like fault can appear at the sole months later, until the fault has grown out.

After cutting holes in the sole, protection is required. There are many proprietary brands but a very effective old form is to cover the sole with Stockholm tar.

Place hair, cut or pulled from your horse's mane or tail, over the Stockholm tar. Layer more Stockholm tar and then a leather pad nailed on under the shoe. This is very effective and hardens the sole.

## Quittor

This is an unusual condition these days as it was commonly seen in draught horses in daily work. It usually appeared as an abscess breaking out at the top of the heel. Conservative treatment seldom works as this is an infection of the lateral cartilage of the pedal bone — sometimes these have turned to bone and fractured, been infected and necrosed. Surgery under local or general anaesthetic involved cutting out the infected/necrotic material and leaving to heal as an open wound (a special knife was designed for this).

## Seedy Toe Surgery

Seedy toe is often a sequel to laminitis or abscess and is an infection running up the inside of the hoof horn, damaging the white line and often then penetrating the sensitive laminae causing pain similar to that of an infection under a human nail.

Surgery entails cutting out all the rotten tissue and the

over-lying horn preferably in a V shape (not an inverted V). An inverted U is also acceptable. The problem with the straight V is difficulty with full drainage and it tends to allow some infection to be left behind.

I remember in 1973, I saw a horse that was three legged lame with seedy toe in both fore hooves and the off hind hoof. Under general anaesthetic, I removed three-quarters of the hoof wall from all three hooves at the one time.

The horse was sore for two months but 12 months later all the hooves were back to normal. Unfortunately, the owner of the horse was found dead in the horse's paddock in 1979, and the horse was finally euthanised by me in 1999 at the age of 30 with no further seedy toe in its life.

# OTHER CONDITIONS

## Snake Bite

Snakes have been given a bad name because if a horse is found dead it is put down to snake bite. I have not seen many examples of truly diagnosed snake bite in horses, although in dogs and cats it is much more prevalent. In the case of the dog and cat, the history is often known and the owners of these animals find their pets frequently with dilated eyes, staggering or generally lazy and flaccid. Obviously, veterinary attention is required to diagnose the correct snake and the administration of correct anti-venom.

In the horse, I suspect not a lot of cases are diagnosed, unless the horse's environment is in a known snake infested area and the vet in the area knows this. I have only diagnosed half a dozen cases. One was a known copperhead bite, one a tiger and four browns. Therefore, I don't claim to be an expert in cases of snake poisoning. However, the copperhead and brown snake symptoms were the same, and the tiger (from a known area) had slightly differing symptoms. Tiger shows a mild colic and a stance similar to a broken pelvis — the horse gently transferring its weight from one hind leg to the other.

Regarding brown/copperheads, in my early days I might have missed a few thinking they were an acute spasmodic colic. Some of these patients lived and others died. However, the symptoms that I have seen have been an exacerbated form of the symptoms of spasmodic colic. The horse will throw itself on the ground, and sometimes immediately get up, then throw itself back down and do this repetitively with little relief from general colic treatment. Often the owner of the horse does not realise the animal has been bitten and can't understand how it could have happened.

Three of my cases have occurred whilst horses were out on a trail or endurance ride. The last was a stabled horse adjacent to the feed shed, possibly near the snake's usual roadway. All these recovered following treatment, with none of the toxic after effects.

## Paterson's Curse (Salvation Jane)

This is a common blue-flowered weed originally brought to Australia from England as a pretty garden plant. Symptoms usually only appear when the condition is advanced. Lethargy and jaundice are the common findings. Diagnosis is by blood test performed by the vet. The weed is extremely abundant and difficult to eradicate. Horses generally do not eat it if there is other feed available. However, some animals do get a taste for it and will seek it out in an addictive manner. Treatment should be provided by your vet.

For prevention the use of a muzzle while the horse is in the paddock is excellent, but the horse needs to be fed twice daily. Muzzles do allow horses to drink.

As a curative diet (if the condition is not too advanced) I advise the feeding of 2 - 4 tablespoons of St Mary's Thistle together with one tablespoon of liquorice root daily. Also, high levels of B group vitamins.

This can be used in an attempt to **prevent** poisoning together with one tablespoon of cotton-seed meal or soya bean meal daily as this contains cystine and methionine — two amino acids protecting the liver.

Other than the above, in cases of prevention and treatment, cut down on other forms of protein like lucerne, beans, lupins etc. Meadow hay and carbohydrates are okay, but not too much carbohydrate if the horse is not in work. Continual availability of hay in the paddock where there is Paterson's Curse is very helpful, if your animal is not muzzled.

**Ergot Poisoning**

This is a black fungus found in wheat, rye grass, oats, hay and fescue. Acute poisoning is not common but I've seen it in the ACT. Acute cases show lesions from lack of circulation in the distal limbs of horses. Lesions are very hard to heal and can progress to gangrene if the horse is not removed from contamination. The ergot found in oats is seen as black on a usually lean oat seed. This seldom leads to the acute form but will cause some low grade gut problems (loose motions or colic) and poor weight gain.

Dr. Richard H Chapman B.V.Sc.

# DOGS AND CATS

## DOGS and CATS

### GENERAL - The Differences

In considering the nature of these animals remember:-

**Cats** are loners in most cases and highly independent in what they do. They even mostly hunt solo, with the exception of the lion.

**Dogs,** on the other hand, are pack animals with a dominant male and female. These keep the pack in a pecking order. If you want your dog to obey you, YOU must be the dominant member of the pack. Your pet will love and respect you more for it, rather than if it is spoilt!

### FEEDING and DIET

Under this section I will touch briefly on diet, because I feel this has a basic effect on gut pathology. What I am about to say is rudimentary and I do not intend to gainsay any dieticians' advice.

I tend to turn to nature for feeds. In the case of dogs and cats, there is a definite trend to feed chicken wings. This I do not comprehend. I look upon diet as that which occurs in nature and there are only *two* wings to a bird. Also a lot of chickens are fed antibiotics in their lifetime and small amounts of these may well be retained in their wings and carcass. There is also little meat on a wing although it does have skin. Surely a natural diet should be similar to nature.

I would therefore suggest:

- **Raw meat on a bone** — chewing and nibbling on meat off the bone massages the gums and keeps the teeth 'brushed' whereas the bone maintains jaw strength and 'spring' in the root system.

- **Skin/fat** — this provides basic vitamins and minerals and is also good exercise for incisor teeth.

- **Offal** — liver especially provides many vitamins specifically vitamin A. In my view, heart, lungs, kidneys and pancreas are less important but the raw pancreas does offer digestive enzymes and it alone is a treatment of pancreatic disease. Of course the Scots use this offal cooked together as 'haggis'!

- **Intestines** — these contain the 'vegetable' section of the diet. Here you have the partially digested green feeds of herbivores with the associated water-soluble vitamins (B group and C). Again I don't expect anyone to feed 'guts' to their pets, but certainly vegetables. Dogs lacking vegetables often eat grass (although some will eat it anyway) and shredded, raw cabbage-type vegetables will often reduce this habit. Cooked vegetables are fine but tend to cause excessive flatulence. Steamed is better so important food factors are not lost.

So in conclusion for dogs' and cats' diets, I say let common sense prevail. The manufacturers of commercial foods take the dietary necessities and incorporate them and indeed add many vitamins and minerals. My remarks above are aimed at those of you who do not want to feed commercial preparations.

# THE MOUTH

These animals naturally feed from the ground and we do indeed usually feed them from bowls at ground level. In nature, these animals feed on their prey. Cats usually consume their prey individually while dogs feed as a pack — with the leader of the pack and the dominant bitch getting the best of the deal — and hence, until age wearies them, they remain the strongest.

Skin, bone, flesh, guts and offal are eaten. The incisor teeth nibble the last of the flesh from the bones, whilst the molars macerate (not grind) the flesh and the large upper and lower molars (carnassial) are used for cracking bone. The eye or canine teeth are *fighting* teeth.

During this process, with mastication mostly being vertical, we see the teeth being cleaned and the gums massaged by the skin and flesh, thus keeping them clean and healthy. Bones are cracked keeping the tooth roots working and the jaw muscles exercised — hence good, healthy teeth.

Nutrients supplied from natural food or prey:

- Skin - minerals and fibre

- Flesh - protein (and high in phosphorous)

- Bones - calcium (and, if large pieces are

swallowed, the vomiting reflex is initiated)

- Guts - vegetables
- Offal - high in vitamin content (especially the liver)

## What do we feed them?

- ○ Processed tinned food - no chewing action half the time
- ○ Popular chicken wings - fat and vitamins in, and under, the skin and probably a lot of fat soluble antibiotics as well.
- ○ Cut-up food - that is maximum one inch squares.
- ○ Bones - some owners feed cooked bones, these can form "concrete" when mixed with faeces and the ensuing constipation takes some relieving. Chop bones and neck bones, especially cooked, are not found on their own in nature in a butchered fashion. These can often get stuck in the intestine and have to be surgically removed.

**Why do they get periodontal disease?** — Inflammation around the tooth base:

From the above, it is obvious; and the prevention should be equally so. In the old days, if an animal died, some country people would give a large part of the carcass to their dog. When he had eaten his fill, as in nature, the rest would be removed and the dog not fed again for a week — think of a wolf pack.

According to the *Guinness Book of Records* book, a dog — a Labrador — fed like this lived to the age of 27 years without the need for false teeth, and a Labrador at that!

Poor teeth and infected gums in dogs and cats lead to toxins escaping into the blood, with the main effect on the kidneys. This, together with an unbalanced ration extra high in protein, accounts for kidney problems in older dogs and cats. Also a prelude to cancer.

I am not saying do not feed biscuits or tinned meat, but I am saying don't do these things exclusively — have a change, say twice a week.

There has been a lot written on the topic of feeding dogs and cats and, of course, there are a vast number of opinions.

Those above are mine and are to make you, the pet-owner, think, think, think.

## ALIMENTARY PROBLEMS

If the animal is obviously ill, you should **contact your veterinarian** as his/her expertise will be required. I can't stress this enough because there can be many causes, some of which will require surgery.

There is also the possibility of dehydration and death if fluids are not given into the vein or under the skin, and of course parvovirus but the dog will then obviously be very sick.

### Diarrhoea

However, diarrhoea (non parvo) is a very common problem, and can often be treated by diet, as in humans. The regimen I have found useful is :

### 5 DAY DIET

**Day 1**: Water at room temperature. If vomiting as well, small portions at a time - may add glucose and can also use broth in place of water.

**Day 2:** May have eggs any way but scrambled, nothing else other than water or broth

**Day 3:** White meat and rice – small portions three or four times daily

**Day 4:** Usual diet - small portions two to four times daily

**Day 5:** Usual diet

## Torsion of the Stomach

This is a condition which is rare but is seen more commonly in the larger breeds of dog (that is Labrador size and up). It occurs when the stomach twists and then blocks the entry point from the oesophagus and the exit point to the small intestine (duodenum).

Symptoms are very rapid and include bloating of the abdomen and attempts by the dog to vomit. In my experience it mostly follows ingestion of a large amount of 'biscuit'.

Surgery is the only treatment for this and if not *immediate* the condition is usually fatal.

A friend of mine had a Great Dane. He is very particular about his dogs and so rang me immediately he noticed the symptoms and I advised him to waste no time in getting the dog to the closest vet. Surgery was commenced within 90 minutes of the onset of symptoms, but the dog still died shortly after surgery.

**Time for the vet at once.**

## Intestinal Parasites

In most cases you will need to consult your vet as they will be up to date with problems in your locality and also with all the latest products. Remember that most puppies and kittens are born with roundworms that have entered via the placenta blood supply.

Your vet will find out if your animal might have the tiny tapeworm *Echinococcus granulosum*, which is the cause of hydatid cysts in humans and other animals.

You can keep up to date when you have animal check ups and/or heartworm treatment and vaccinations.

You can also, of course, try the five day diet (as above) if the dog is not obviously ill.

# COUGHS and COLDS

## DOGS

A cough is a symptom not a disease. If a cough persists it is probably worth a visit to your vet as it is a manifestation of one or some of the following:

- A throat scratch, from a stick or something like that
- Mild inflammation of the throat
- Foreign body, stuck in the throat
- A virus like kennel cough, which will usually clear itself in 7 - 21 days, symptoms do upset owners — so why not vaccinate?
- Tonsillitis
- Heart problems - usually older dogs;
- Infections, such as pneumonia, bronchitis or even migrating parasites

A 'cold', such as a runny nose, is not common and usually relates to a foreign body, like a grass seed. Can be viral or post viral involving a sinus. In old dogs rotten teeth can also be the cause.

**CATS**

Common causes are:

- Cat flu - includes weeping eyes
- Post flu sinusitis
- Tooth root infections
- Parasites – cough only

**All these indicate a visit to your vet.**

## EYES and EARS

**EYES**

Stating the obvious, an animal has two eyes which are both delicate structures. The loss of one, therefore, is serious, the loss of *both* is disastrous with the possible exception of the dog, which can survive when blind due to its extra good sense of smell and familiarity with its surroundings.

Do not hesitate to contact your vet even if you consider the condition harmless. Without going into the complete anatomy of the eye I would like to comment on the pupil because this is a useful guide to your vet when you ring him/her.

- **Dilated pupil** – in our species the dilated pupil is always round, and when fully dilated leaves the iris as a narrow band surrounding the black-looking pupil. This occurs naturally in the dark, and as the surroundings get light, so the pupil constricts (gets smaller).

- **Constricted pupil** – in bright daylight the pupil is at its maximum constriction (smallest).

Here there is a species difference:

**DOGS** — the pupil remains round. In nature the dog requires all-round vision but not so much lateral vision, as it hunts in packs and generally wants to see what is in front of it.

**CATS** — these animals are stalkers and therefore have tunnel vision. Their constricted pupil is vertical so they can see up and down whilst stalking their prey.

## Conditions owners are likely to take lightly

Weepy eyes in dogs and cats are not often a problem, but can occasionally be caused by in-growing eyelashes, lids turned in or out, an early ulcer on the eyeball or other deeper problems — so don't dismiss it.

## Eye Preparations

Available, without prescription, from the pharmacy are Brolene eye drops or ointment, or Antistine Privine eye drops, which can help alleviate discomfort until the vet sees your animal. Antibiotic and atropine eye preparations are available from your veterinarian or on prescription from the pharmacy. All commercial eye drops/ointments are provided as sterile products but any unused portion is to be discarded after 28 days.

**On no account use preparations containing cortisone of any type** unless prescribed by your veterinarian for the current condition. Do not use any left-over corticosteroid preparations.

Sometimes, particularly after extended antibiotic use, an

ulcer can become infected by fungus. This is extremely serious and, therefore, if the ulcer being treated has not responded well and is mostly becoming more yellow, your vet will need to *see* the animal again and take a swab for microscopic examination.

## UNDER EYES

The nictitating membrane, or third eyelid, is well developed in reptiles and acts like the eyelids in mammals. This is far less developed in mammals.

Conditions seen in:

## DOGS:

Very rarely a problem. Occasionally tumours are seen. In brachiocephalic dogs like bulldogs, boxers, pugs, etc, a condition called cherry eye occurs, whereby the cartilage in the membrane curls and causes a cherry like lesion in the inside corner of the eye. Your vet will treat this condition surgically.

## CATS:

Mostly seen as coming up to halfway across the eyeball, this can be produced by putting pressure on the eyeball, which depresses the fat behind the eyeball and causes the membrane to slide across the eye.

This also occurs if the fat behind the eyeball is reduced in cases of systemic disease, or even a hairball in the stomach. Sometimes with corneal damage when the muscles behind the eyeball contract with the pain of the ulcer.

This condition is seldom serious, unless it doesn't resolve itself in 7 - 10 days when veterinary help should be sought.

## EAR CONDITIONS

## DOGS:

If your dog suddenly starts shaking its head, rubbing its ears along the ground or scratching the ear madly and tilting its head, you can bet your bottom dollar there is a grass seed, fly, or foreign body in there.

If it lasts more than half an hour, it won't be a fly and the dog will need an anaesthetic to get the thing out — vet job.

## HORMONAL CONDITIONS

**DOGS -** hormonal imbalances usually require veterinary treatments.

**Adrenal imbalance** — Cushing's Disease

**Thyroid imbalance** — weight gain and bilateral flank baldness.

Fat bitches that were spayed before puberty respond well with oestrogen treatments, both in energy and loss of weight.

There is an old saying: 'let a bitch have a litter before desexing and she'll never get fat'. In the old days, when a bitch came into season she'd get in whelp, and this, of course, would happen in the first season. These bitches seldom got fat when desexed later.

Therefore, I tend to go against the modern line of many vets and prefer not to desex prior to the first season, as I feel that reaching puberty and spaying 3 months after the first season, tends to reduce the change of obesity.

You also see that many plump young girls will become a different shape after puberty!

**CATS** - the commonest hormonal deficiency is seen in male neutered cats and presents as a balding of the inner thighs and belly and sometimes the back. This is also commoner when the cat has been desexed younger than 6 months. This responds well to veterinary treatment.

In the older cat, weight loss is very common and is often due to kidney disease, but, too much thyroid can also be the problem. Weight issues are therefore for your vet to sort out.

# TRAINING

New techniques, advice, etc are continually coming up. I am only giving two techniques for this, two or three to stop dogs jumping up on you, plus one for stopping them chewing your hand.

Firstly, it is obviously normal for your pet to perform its **bodily functions**, but not normal for it to immediately know where. Thus it performs when it needs to.

It is therefore, no good to scold, smack the animal or to rub its nose in it, before simply throwing the animal outside. Next time it's going to be more wary and try to hide it. *And* it will get more and more ingenious.


## HOUSE TRAINING

1.    The first method is this:

Collect half or some of the excrement and take it outside. You then show the animal what it has done inside and scold or smack it.

Immediately, take the animal out and show it the urine (probably on paper) or faeces outside. Now praise it and give it a treat.

Next time don't do this just once but three times:

   •    inside (scold) – outside (praise)

- inside – outside
- inside – outside.

At the next indiscretion, increase the inside-outside number of repetitions.

I have never seen his method take longer than three days and often only one day.

2.   The alternative is to put the animal out after every feed, because this is the most common time for their toiletries, and praise them when they perform.

Likewise, if you catch them performing, put them out straight away.

This perhaps is the most common method used today.

**JUMPING UP**

Dogs jumping up can be annoying.

- Once again salt and sugar treatment. Should the dog jump up – squeeze its paws hard – it winces and goes down – now praise the dog.

- An easier method is to tread on its back foot every time it jumps up and then praise the dog when it is back down with all four feet on the ground.

## HAND CHEWING

- If a pup is always chewing your hand, don't take the hand away but push it down the pup's throat and make it gag for 10 or so seconds! I've found this foolproof.

These methods were taught to me by an exceptionally good remedial dog trainer in England with whom I had many dealings and who was an excellent client of mine. He was a trainer of police dogs and expert in the rehabilitation of vicious dogs.

## MUSCULO-SKELETAL

This perhaps is the hardest thing to describe and tell you what to do about it. Diagnosis is the most important and most difficult part of it.

Once again **this is a veterinary domain**. Short of the obvious cut or sore paw, diagnosis is the game.

Breed incidence of various conditions are known to your veterinarian, including such things as:

- Hip dysplasia

- Elbow dysplasia

- Stifle ligaments - internal and external

- Displaced tibial crest

Should your dog break its femur (thigh bone) the usual treatment is surgery to pin the fracture.

If you cannot afford this, most people are told to euthanase the dog as it is in pain.

On many occasions, when the owner cannot afford the surgery, I have told them to keep the animal confined and I usually give it some support, that is Elastoplast or plaster of Paris/fibreglass.

In four to six months the fracture has healed albeit the leg is shorter. Surgery can also have its problems such as

© 2015 R. H. Chapman

non union of the bone and poor wound healing.

I have used this method only for people who won't or can't afford pinning.

It started in 1962, when I was a young graduate practising in Orbost, Victoria. A large Mastiff cross sustained a mid-shaft fracture of the femur. The dog belonged to my neighbour who was a local 'cocky' and did not believe in spending money on dogs. 'She'll be right' he said and six months later the dog was absolutely okay.

The latest was in 2008, when a friend's Jack Russell got a lower femur fracture. The owner was unable to contain the dog, nor would it keep on any support. In four months, the Jack Russell was fine and the x-ray confirmed bone union.

I have had several other successes and no failures!


**Arthritis** is very common in dogs — less diagnosed in cats.

This can affect all joints including those of the spine. There are a myriad of drugs for treatment of this condition and your vet will know which drugs to prescribe.

**RESTRAINTS** - Used for biting or vicious animals.

## Dogs

Obviously muzzle to prevent biting, but sometimes they have to be restrained to get these on, or to hold them still afterwards or to inject with a sedative etc.

Position yourself behind the dog, and in the case of a large dog, straddle it. Place the thumbs behind the collar and grab the scruff of the neck with your fingers in front of the collar leaving the thumbs behind. The collar acts like an anchor so the dog can't turn its head.

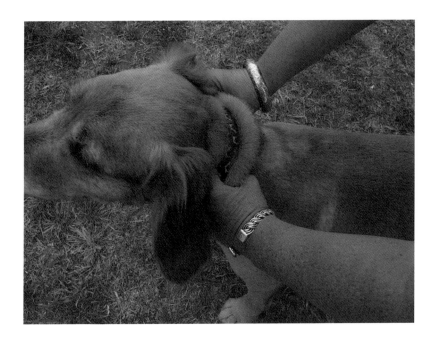

© 2015 R. H. Chapman

Another way is to use a 'dog catcher'.

This is a hollow tube or pipe, with a loop passed through the pipe. Alternately, one end of the rope is attached to one end of the pipe and the other end passed through the pipe. Both of these form a noose at one end of the pipe.

Loop the noose over the animal's head and pull tight. The head is then kept a pole length away and may be pushed against the wall or the floor for extra leverage.

This method is not practical for home use generally, but a ring placed permanently in the floor or wall may be used. Pass the lead through the ring and draw the animals head up tight to it.

Note: this will fail if the collar is too loose. It is a common failing amongst dog owners to have the collar too loose so the dog can 'slip it'. (Should be as tight as detachable collars on shirts — old men will remember these!)

**Cats**

- The easiest way is "Mum's way". Hold the cat tightly by the scruff and it will have difficulty in reaching you – even with its back legs. If it tries, you can hold its legs and stretch the animal out – but be firm.

- Wrap the cat in a towel or blanket with the head

out. Keep the wrapping tight around the neck to prevent the front paws getting out to scratch you.

- If the cat is hissing at you – a spray of water in the face will stop it for long enough for someone to grab it.

Note - most dogs and cats do not need these methods of restraint.

# SKIN

There are numerous causes of skin disease in dogs and cats. Most, if not all, require the attention of your veterinarian, because, as in humans, diseases of the skin are the most difficult to cure. Few if any are lethal – various treatments can be found at the end of this section.

**Ringworm - t**here are two types:

- *Microsporum* - small lesions
- *Trichophyton*

Besides treating the animal, you must treat coats and bedding.

Cats may often have ringworm without showing signs. Usually the first hint is that a member of the family comes down with it. Diagnosis of the animal is done by your vet.

Dogs and cats can be treated orally with a prescription drug called **griseofulvin** as well as topically with washes.

## Anal glands

Itching under the tail is often thought to be due to worms, but is often due to **anal glands** or 'skunk glands'. These are situated at 4 and 8 o'clock, a little below the anus and about 3mm — 5mm deep, and are actually sacs.

Signs of impaction are 'skating' along the ground in an effort to expel the contents. Sometimes dogs may be lying perfectly peacefully and will suddenly get up and shoot into a corner, they may even yelp.

If the impaction is not alleviated, usually by your vet, it will eventually form a very painful abscess, usually one side being greater than the other. Hence, if you see this 'skating' or any of the symptoms above, don't assume worms, call your vet.

You can learn how to express these glands yourself. But be careful, because it is very easy to get a face full of very smelly product!

## Ectoparasites — under skin

### Dogs

- Ear mites (otodectes)
- Demodectic mites (follicle)
- Sarcoptic mites (burrowing)
- Fleas
- Lice
- Ticks
- Flies

**Ear mites** — are common in dogs and cats as well. Cats are less affected than dogs and therefore can provide a latent source of infection if you have both a cat and dog. These mites have a life cycle of egg to adult of about 3 weeks. The mites build up a black discharge in the ear, which can be so thick that it hinders treatment. This needs to be cleaned before treatment applications.

Treatment consists of cleaning the ear which can be done with 1% hydrogen peroxide, a wax solvent and any sort of oil. Treatment into the ear with a mitocide (which you can get from your vet) is then carried out. Most directions say 2 - 6 drops but I usually just flood the ear, and give it a good massage around the base. I do this once daily for a week, then twice weekly for 6 weeks, even if the ear looks clean and there are no symptoms. This procedure usually kills all of the mites. It is a good idea for you to let your vet have a look at the ears at least at the start of the treatment, as they will give you the latest treatment advice.

Complications — why I suggest you see your vet early is to try to avoid complications, and to give you a true diagnosis. Some times with these ear mites, the dog will scratch its ear so hard that it bursts a blood vessel in the earflap, causing it to swell into an enormous blood blister The dog will hold its head to the side and also shake its head. If you leave this alone it will in time cure itself, but the ear will shrivel and crinkle and leave a 'cauliflower' ear. Surgery by your vet can alleviate this and stop the ear from shrivelling.

**Fleas** — these can cause an allergic dermatitis. Usually it is not difficult to find fleas, if you can't see them you can see 'flea dirt', which looks like black dirt in the coat — commonly seen near the back above the tail. If you put this dirt in water it turns red. When a dog is highly sensitised to fleas, one bite will cause acute irritation, especially near the tail. In these cases you are unlikely to find fleas or flea dirt. Hence a visit to your vet is probably necessary.

Treatment and prevention - there are many 'pour on' and 'spot on' treatments, which you can try, but a phone call to your vet is the most sensible course, as they will be able to give you the best advice for the location you are in. You will also get advice as to other precautions you can take such as killing the larvae. Flea pupae (cocoons) can lie dormant for many years. Vibrations will cause them to hatch.

An anecdote regarding this is the case of a 'haunted house', in Kent, England. The house had been empty for over 20 years. Eventually, when it became part of a

© 2015 R. H. Chapman

deceased's estate, it was put up for sale. With much trepidation the realtor in charge of its sale entered the house. Within a matter of minutes he was crawling with fleas! This gives you an idea of the dormancy of the pupa : the vibration caused them to hatch.

**Mange** - this condition is caused by mites -

- Follicular (in the hair follicles) - **demodex**
- Burrowing - **sarcops**

Diagnosis of this is via a skin scraping, which your vet would undertake.

> **Demodectic mange** can be present at birth where it is probably also common in the Dachshund or Doberman breeds. This is usually in the form of a thin coat, especially ears and nose. It does not seem to worry the dog and may go undiagnosed through life. The acute form looks nasty, as the affected areas erupt into a pustular form which is not affected by antibiotics on their own. This used to be difficult to treat effectively and permanently, but now with the advent of ivermectin the position has changed.

> At present mange needs vet attention as washes are mostly ineffective.

> **Sarcoptic mange** - commonly seen in the belly,

in the groin and armpits. This is red and itchy. Part of the treatment is to make sure the bedding is washed in very hot water and preferably medicated when the dog is washed. Once again, ivermectin is a good veterinary treatment, but washes are also good. It would be advisable to get veterinary input for control and treatment.

**Lice** — these present as slow moving or stationary white objects. The eggs are glued to the hair and are only removed with difficulty. Treatment is simple as insecticidal washes are very effective. In order to kill any eggs that may hatch it is advisable to give weekly washes for 4 - 6 weeks.

**Ticks** — in certain areas of Australia these will cause paralysis and death in dogs. Coastal areas are more prone to ticks.

When a tick gets on a dog it is very small and usually goes unnoticed. It takes its time to attach and when it does it harpoons its tongue into the skin. I say harpoon because that is what the tongue is like. It then injects its saliva to help it suck blood and this saliva holds the poison.

The body of the tick gradually swells as it fills with blood until it gets to the size of a small Malteser, the tick is now sated and will fall off. If this happens without you even noticing it, it will help give your dog an immunity. How nice.

However, a dog with no immunity would be showing 'the wobbles' in the hind limbs as probably the first symptom you would notice.

If you live on the coast or, even more important, if you have returned with your dog from a stint at the coast and even when you are at the coast, examine your dog all over, daily. Areas you are likely to find ticks are where the dog can't get them off by itself, occasionally between the toes and rarely inside the prepuce or vagina. In one instance I've seen it just inside the lip.

When you find a tick don't just pull it out, as you will leave the harpoon tongue inside and this in due course will fester, but you will have removed the chance of further toxins. If you squeeze the body when trying to do this you may cause more toxins to enter the body.

The easiest way to remove a tick is to apply a glowing cigarette, or some form of heat, to the body of the tick. The tick will withdraw its tongue and be easy to pick off, if it doesn't fall off.

Next best thing is to use forceps and hold the head below the body, rock and pull and try to ease the harpoon tongue out. Vets do this very well. Another method is to cover the tick with oil or grease, like Vaseline, right down to the skin level of the animal. This will in turn suffocate and kill the tick, so it will retract its harpoon and fall off. This is a slow process and may allow more toxins into your dog. If your dog is staggering go straight to the vet, otherwise just keep an eye on them and keep looking for more ticks.

**Prevention** — talk to your vet before heading off for your coastal break, as the vet is the right person to advise you on this. These days there are excellent oral preventions lasting from 1 to 4 months. So you should be able to prevent very expensive veterinary treatment.


## Non-Parasitic Balding

Atopic balding is a non specific condition, with irritation, that needs to be diagnosed by your vet, who will treat it with an expensive drug called Cyclosporin.

However, before going to this extent you can try these old-fashioned treatments:

- Vitamin A supplementation plus some yellow sulphur, but just a pinch daily in the feed.

- Grinding up poplar seeds and making into an ointment using organic honey. This is somewhat messy and the animal will probably try to lick it off – but I have seen it work.

- Chilblain ointment, which contains niacin

(nicotinic acid), can also be used in conjunction with tablet form. This increases blood supply to extremities and the skin, and I've had most success with Chihuahuas and Dachshunds.

# WOUNDS

Treatment of wounds is very much up to the individual and that includes veterinarians. I am, therefore, not going into a lot of detail on every aspect of wound healing and treatment, but just give a few tips to try and reduce the cost and prolongation of treatment.

## Burns

Treatment is of course related to severity — some require euthanasia and most require veterinary care.

However, as an initial treatment I use cold water (if early), and mixtures containing organic (untreated) honey. This includes a honey mix with such things as Ungvita cream (vitamin A), yoghurt (natural, preferably home made) or anything that is solar protective.

## Cuts and Abrasions

Cold hose first if you can. Many of these of course need suturing. What I am now telling you, can be done as a first aid measure whilst considering calling a vet, or waiting for their arrival.

To **staunch bleeding**, apply as many spider webs as you can find over the wound, and then pressure bandage if that is possible (pressure bandaging cannot be done on the body or high up on the limbs).

© 2015 R. H. Chapman

The bandage should start above or below the wound, whichever way is best, to push the skin over the lesion.

On the body you seldom find a wound that causes severe bleeding so in these cases you can usually await treatment by a vet.

The old remedy was to throw a handful of lime over the wound and let the animal get on with it.

**Cut type wound**s in dogs and cats are usually easy to wrap when they occur in the limbs, especially the more bloody wounds in the paw region. Most small animal wounds are easy to suture.

In all species, **wounds near the eye** should be seen **by a vet** — most especially those affecting the eyelid margins.

Any damage in that area may well cause some dysfunction of the lid, thus leaving part of the eye uncovered when blinking and hence causing some drying out and chronic ulcer formation.

Alternatively, the eyelid may turn in slightly causing the eyelashes to irritate the surface of the eyeball. Therefore, call the vet or take the animal to the clinic.

# APPENDICES

# RICHARD'S RECIPES FOR HORSES

## MASHES

### Basic Bran Mash
    1.5kg bran
    2 to 3 tablespoons salt
    2 to 3 handfuls crushed oats
    4 to 5 litres boiling water
Place solids in 10 litre bucket, add water and stir.
Cover and leave 20 to 30minutes to cook.
Stir after 40 minutes, and make sure it is not too hot to feed.

### Purgative Bran Mash
As above, but add to the water :
    half a kilogram of Epsom salts and
    1 kilogram of sugar.
Boil and add to above.

For a tricky horse, cover either of the above with **crushed oats and molasses.**

### Bran and oatmeal
Basic bran mash with 2 to 4 handfuls of coarse pinhead (fine) oatmeal (tasty and nutritive)

**Basic Linseed Mash**
Maximum of 250g linseed
Place into 5 litres of water.
Boil vigorously for 15 minutes while stirring and simmer for 4 to 6 hours.
Feed the lot including the mucilage, and what is uneaten goes rancid quickly, so throw it away.
Give this for a maximum of twice a week or till the horse's faeces tend to soften. This is a good tonic and used for horses with a poor appetite.

**Convalescing Mashes**
**For digestive and parasitic conditions**
Basic bran and linseed mashes. Make separately and mix together.

**For anorexia and debilitation**
**Basic bran mash and barley**
Soak barley for 6 hours and boil for half an hour, or just boil the barley for 2 hours. Make separately and mix in equal proportions.

**For anorexia and debilitation. Also for a change, or if the horse is dehydrated.**
Basic bran mash or **barley plus succulents**
Add to bran or barley mashes — carrots, swedes, apples, parsnips

**For very sick horse (with intestinal trouble following diarrhoea)**
Basic bran mash with well boiled porridge 3:1 or 2:1

**Additions to all mashes if required**
Wash dandelion leaves and roots, lucern or other green food.
Crushed ivy leaves on top

**For sick horse**
Well-boiled kipper including the water it was boiled in.
If not eaten in 2 to 3 hours, discard.

**Remember** — if a mash is too hot, it burns the horse's nose and that animal will never touch another mash again.

## POULTICES FOR HORSES

**Bread** — useful if camping or trekking. Boil the billy can with lots of salt added, add to bread to make it soggy but not runny. Put the poultice on neat. Bandage, or put in a sanitary towel with padding removed.

Horses will like to eat this as salty bread is quite tasty. If you have any Epsom salts, this is better as it doesn't taste as good.

**Bran** — as for bread but using bran instead. Epsom salts are good, salt and sugar are good too, but you may have to muzzle the horse.

**Cabbage** — cut and cook till soggy, may add salts as above.

**Proprietary** — there are many such as kaolin, Antiphlogistine and Animalintex.

**Iodine and sugar**

**Soap and sugar**

# ALTERNATIVE TREATMENTS

For those intent on using natural therapies.

Below are the treatments I have tried and found to work, but as in anything, not 100% of the time. No homeopathic treatment should be used alongside cortisone.

**Aconite 30C**.

- **Reticence in Floating**: 1 when needed, then leave 10 to 15 minutes and try to float.

- Also aids in reluctance to go into racing barriers.

- Works if fear is the problem.

**Arnica 30C**          1 three times daily for **bruising**

**Arnica 200C**

- pre-operatively and post-operatively.

- Aids in **trauma** (worked on me with shoulder surgery)

**Belladonna 6C**      1 six times on the 1st day only for **fever**

**Aconite 6C**      as for Belladonna above

**Bellis Perennis 30C**

> For **bruising 48 hours old** 1 x three times daily for 3 days

**Hekla Lava 30C to 200C**

> For bony lesions,
>
> hip dysplasia,
>
> **arthritis alleviation** not cure

**Carb Fluor 30C**      as above for *Hekla lava*

**Hypericum** cream **wounds and ulcers**

**Calendula** lotion      **wounds and ulcers**

**Ignatia M**      1 a week for **separation, pining**

**Ledum pal 30C**      1 two or three x daily for **puncture wounds**

**Rhus tox M**      1 x weekly for 4 weeks **sore back**

> **NB** if used on a horse, check saddle first

**Rhus tox 200C**      1 daily for **joint pain** especially cold, windy weather.

Also **allergic itch**

**Ruta grav 200C**      1 twice daily for **tendons and ligaments** — especially suspensory

**Selenica 30C**      1 three x daily for **chronic founder**

**Selenica 200C scar tissue**      1 weekly for 12 weeks for **scars and scar tissue**

**Thuja 200C & M**

- For **sarcoids** (about 25% successful) **200C** 1 x daily early on, then **M** 1 x weekly
- Warts/papillomatosis will go on their own within 3 months.

## MISCELLANEOUS ITEMS

**Kerosene** – this is an old bush treatment for most infectious conditions and others.

1.    Pink eye in cattle - conjunctivitis, will sting a lot and can do damage.

2.    Any wound together with a handful of lime, or else lime on its own.

3.    Over the coat for external parasite treatment, including bot eggs. However is very caustic to cats and nearly as much to dogs.

**Stomach tubing** – this is the vets job. Some horsemen feel they are capable, but for legal reasons should only do this for their own horses. For dogs and cats it's done under anaesthetic. In the horse a long necked bottled is best for drenching. If the liquid is bland, add the juice of 1 or 2 lemons, which will help the swallowing reflex. In dogs and cats a syringe is best used, the use of lemon juice is also appropriate.

### EAR Recipes

Pour **methylated spirit** in the ear. After the animal has stopped going crazy, put a little boracic into the ear – for **EMERGENCY USE ONLY.**

**Recipe for Fly Ears**:

Melt a moth ball or naphthalene flakes together with camphor.

Mix with tea tree oil.

Allow to cool to an ointment.

N.B. Specific quantities are not essential even if the end result is more like a lotion.

## Acknowledgements:

To my wife, Jan, who did all the early typing and editing.

To my associate, Dr Rochelle Prattley, and many of my clientele who have been pushing me to get this done.

To my sister, Marion Eaton, who finally pulled this book together after I had been fiddling about for 10 years!

And to Annabel Dobson for her encouragement and help.

Thank you all.

Lightning Source UK Ltd.
Milton Keynes UK
UKIC02n2149210217
294971UK00001B/3